OBSTETRICS AND GYNECOLOGY ADVANCES

CONTRACEPTION

UNMET NEEDS, EXISTING OPTIONS, AND NEW TECHNOLOGIES

OBSTETRICS AND GYNECOLOGY ADVANCES

Additional books in this series can be found on Nova's website under the Series tab.

Additional e-books in this series can be found on Nova's website under the e-book tab.

OBSTETRICS AND GYNECOLOGY ADVANCES

CONTRACEPTION

UNMET NEEDS, EXISTING OPTIONS, AND NEW TECHNOLOGIES

ALICIA Y. ARMSTRONG
EDITOR

New York

For permission to use material from this book please contact us:
Telephone 631-231-7269; Fax 631-231-8175
Web Site: http://www.novapublishers.com

Library of Congress Cataloging-in-Publication Data

ISBN: 978-1-63482-145-2
Library of Congress Control Number: 2015931764

Published by Nova Science Publishers, Inc. † New York

Contents

Preface		**vii**
Chapter 1	Unmet Needs *Mae Wu Healy, DO, Karenne Fru, MD, PhD and Alicia Armstrong, MD, MHSCR*	**1**
Chapter 2	Existing Contraceptive Options *Matthew Connell, MD, Tiffany Hailstorks, MD and Nneoma Nwachuku, MD*	**39**
Chapter 3	Contraception: New Technologies *Nicole Banks, MD and Diana Blithe, PhD*	**91**
Index		**121**

Preface

In this book, the authors review a number of topics in this important subject area. In the section on unmet needs, the authors review the unmet needs for contraception in the U.S., UK, Europe, Asia and the developing world as well as unmet needs in special populations such as adolescents, women with medical conditions and women living with HIV. The authors review the current options for contraception with special emphasis on efficacy, side effects and patient selection and identify gaps in contraception options. Finally, the authors review some of the latest advances and innovations in contraceptive technology.

Chapter 1 – The goal of this chapter is to highlight the key problems of unmet contraceptive needs and contextualize them with the aim of making clear the areas for improvement. While great strides have been made in generating contraceptive medications, devices and procedures, the fact remains that not every woman who desires or could benefit from contraception is using it. As much attention has been paid to global unmet contraceptive needs, this chapter briefly touches on the global problem but focuses instead on the medical, cultural and economic reasons for unmet contraceptive needs in the United States in particular.

Chapter 2 – An estimated 41% of pregnancies are unintended. Globally, 86 million pregnancies were unintended. These unintended pregnancies resulted in 41 million abortions, 33 million unplanned births and 11 million in miscarriages. Nearly half of all pregnancies in the U.S. are unintended, which is defined as any pregnancy either mistimed, unplanned or unwanted. Safe effective contraception is clearly one of the most important areas of reproductive health for women. In this chapter the authors will review the current options for contraception, with special emphasis on efficacy, side effects and patient selection and identify gaps in contraception options.

Chapter 3 – Despite significant improvements in contraceptive options, there continues to be a high rate of unplanned pregnancy. About half of these pregnancies occur in contraceptive users, largely due to inconsistent or incorrect use. This fact points to a significant unmet need for effective and reliable male and female contraception. Development of new contraceptive options for women is focused on meeting the following goals: decreasing the risks of current hormonal contraception and improving compliance with easier to use methods such as a transdermal patch, vaginal ring or long-acting reversible contraception options. New programs are needed to explore non-hormonal methods targeting molecules involved in ovulation, fertilization and implantation, and to identify options that have additional health benefits, such as prevention of sexually transmitted disease. Current male contraception options are limited to condoms and vasectomy; however, studies demonstrate that male hormonal contraception could be an effective option for the future. Additional research into non-hormonal approaches to testicular or epididymal targets necessary for sperm production or function may result in effective products for male contraception. Future contraceptive research and development should continue to address the above listed goals, as well as expand access to reliable contraception both within the United States and globally.

In: Contraception
Editor: Alicia Y. Armstrong
ISBN: 978-1-63482-145-2

Chapter 1

Unmet Needs

Mae Wu Healy, DO, Karenne Fru MD, PhD and Alicia Armstrong MD, MHSCR* [*]
Program in Reproductive and Adult Endocrinology, Eunice Kennedy Shriver National Institute of Child Health and Human Development, National Institutes of Health, Bethesda, MD, US

Abstract

The goal of this chapter is to highlight the key problems of unmet contraceptive needs and contextualize them with the aim of making clear the areas for improvement. While great strides have been made in generating contraceptive medications, devices and procedures, the fact remains that not every woman who desires or could benefit from contraception is using it.

As much attention has been paid to global unmet contraceptive needs, this chapter briefly touches on the global problem but focuses instead on the medical, cultural and economic reasons for unmet contraceptive needs in the United States in particular.

[*] Corresponding author: Alicia Armstrong, Armstroa@mail.nih.gov.

Introduction: Overview of Global Unmet Needs

Globally, the unmet contraception need cannot be overstated [1]. This problem has been extensively studied in developing countries where access is often the primary etiologic factor [2]. In some developed countries, like the United States, high-unintended pregnancy rates persist despite access to modern contraceptive methods [3,4]. In this section we will briefly review global unmet contraceptive needs with a focus on unmet contraceptive needs in the United States.

Early data demonstrating unmet contraceptive needs came from survey studies carried out in developing countries in the 1960s[5]. These "KAP" surveys asked women about *K*nowledge of, *A*ttitudes towards, *P*ractice of birth control, in addition to family size preference. The results showed that a substantial number of women who wished to cease childbearing were not using contraception, illustrating the gap between their reproductive intentions and their actual use of contraception [6]. These women were thus termed "KAP-Gap" [7,8] which was replaced in 1978 by the currently used term "unmet need" [9].

The phrase "unmet need" has been used to describe the misuse or lack of use of contraception and the role it plays in unwanted or unplanned pregnancies. The term includes women with an unmet need for limiting, defined as no further desire for future children, but who are not using contraception. It also describes those who have an unmet need for spacing, described as wishing to postpone another birth yet are not using any birth control methods [10]. There are a number of reasons for a lack of contraceptive use including financial, cultural and religious issues. These reasons may supersede a woman's perceived risk of pregnancy and subsequent childcare.

That said, there has been great progress in meeting the contraceptive needs of married women in the reproductive ages over the past four decades [11]. This progress is central to the United Nations Millennium Development Goal of improving maternal health [12]. Worldwide, as of 2012, the unmet need for contraception among women in the developing world is estimated to range from 221 to 222 million [1,13]. It has been predicted that if all the unmet needs for these women were fulfilled, 54 million unintended pregnancies each year could be prevented [13]. The increased contraceptive use in developing nations is mainly attributed to increased access to care [1]. There remain, however, areas such as Sub-Saharan Africa and South Asia that continue to lag in their progression toward addressing unmet needs. This is largely due to poor investment by national governments and agencies leading to continued limited access to care for reproductive aged women living in these countries. [12, 14]

Despite efforts to increase modern contraceptive use, traditional methods of contraception are still being practiced. Traditional methods, defined as either withdrawal or periodic abstinence, are also considered unmet need given their inconsistent application and unreliability in preventing pregnancy [11,14]. Globally, 32% of currently married women are using a form of modern contraception and 11% are using traditional methods[14]. Between the years of 1990 and 2010, global contraceptive prevalence among married women, or those in a relationship between the ages of 15-49, had increased from 54.8% to 63.3% [1]. Accordingly, the unmet need for family planning decreased from 15.4% in 1990 to 12.3% in 2010[1]. This continues to translate to a significant number of women in their reproductive age worldwide who had unmet needs in 2010. If women users of traditional methods are included in these numbers, the unmet need for all methods around the world increases from 146 to 221 million women [1]. Estimates of the total demand for contraception, inclusive of women currently using methods and women with unmet needs were about 900 million in 2010. Projecting into the year 2015 using these numbers and trends (Figure 1), estimates of the total demand would rise to 962 million women. The total number of contraceptive users would increase from 753 to 808 million women. The unmet needs of users, not inclusive of traditional methods users, increases from 146 million to 153 million. If we include women currently using traditional methods, there would be an estimated 233 million women increased from 221 million with an unmet need for modern methods [1].

Specifically in the United States, despite better access to contraception, there still exists significant unmet need [15]. Financial costs, religious or cultural biases and lack of fundamental knowledge about how contraception works and the benefits it may carry play a much larger role for women in the U.S., where access is greatly expanded. The remaining barriers to contraception can be categorized as issues at the level of the patient, the provider, or the infrastructure of the health care system. Twenty-nine percent of patients cited fear of adverse effects or general health concerns with contraceptive use, making it the most common reason for lack of use [14]. The next most common reasons cited by 18% of women, included infrequent intercourse, pregnancy related reasons such as breastfeeding, or opposition from the husband and/or family. There are also significant identified barriers at the provider level such as lack of knowledge leading to poor counseling, lack of necessary skills in techniques such as intrauterine device insertion, misconceived notions about certain contraceptives like long-acting reversible contraception (LARC), and poor management of adverse effects [16-18]. In addition to these challenges, health care system barriers include poor financial resources, geographic inaccessibility, and inadequate human resources and support [19].

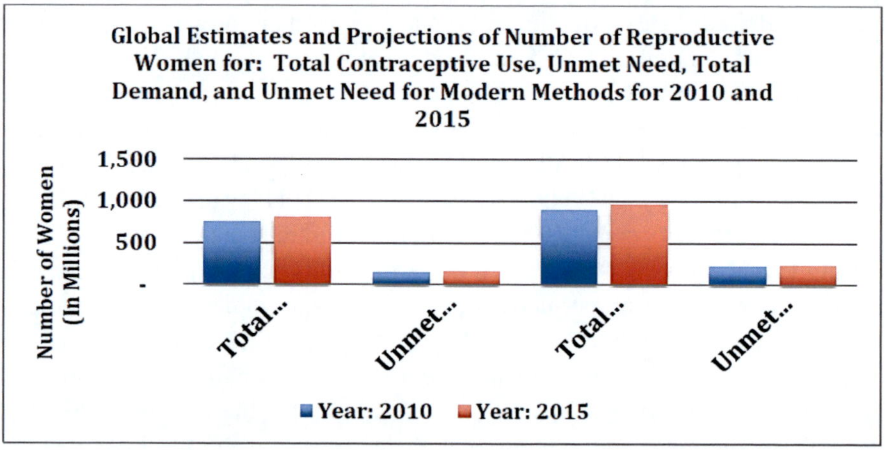

Figure generated with data from: Alkema L, Kantorova V, Menozzi C, Biddlecom A. *Lancet*. 381,1642 (2013).

Figure 1. Total contraceptive use refers to any form of contraception, including modern and traditional methods. Total demand refers to the combined number of total contraceptive use and unmet need. Unmet need for modern methods refers to the number of unmet need and those using traditional methods.

Unmet Needs in the United States

In the United States, approximately 50% of all pregnancies are unintended [20]. These pregnancy rates are higher among young women and adolescent groups, certain ethnic/racial minority groups and those with lower levels of education and income [21]. The Department of Health and Human Services has made it a goal to reduce the national level of unintended pregnancy. It is estimated to cost taxpayers approximately $11.1 billion dollars each year for unintended pregnancies (Figure 2), a substantial financial burden [22].

Conversely, there are 38.4 million women between the ages of 15 and 44 years using contraception, according to the United States National Survey of National Growth [23]. The most common method used among 47.3% of married couples is permanent sterilization; 30.2% tubal occlusion and 17.1% vasectomy [24]. The number of tubal ligations over time has remained fairly stable since the 1970s. The rate peaked at over 702,000 procedures in 1977, remained stable through the next 2 decades, and has since decreased slightly to 643,000 in 2006 [25]. In comparison to permanent sterilization, 18.6% of couples use oral contraceptives, 15.3% use male condoms, 7.1% use intrauterine devices and 3.9% use injectable contraceptives (Figure 3) [26].

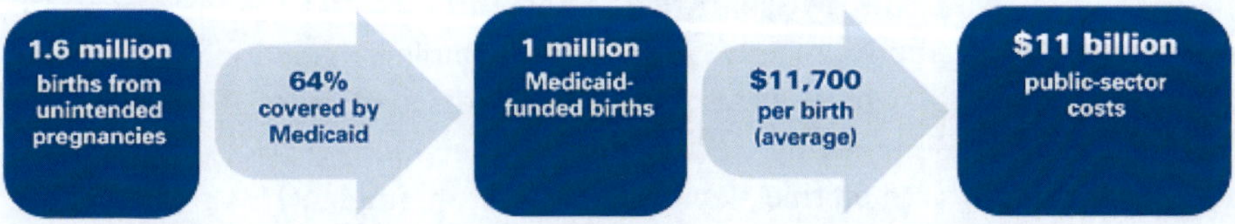

Source: Gold RB, Wise investment: reducing the steep cost to Medicaid of unintended pregnancy in the United States, Guttmacher Policy Review, 2011, 14(3):6–10, Figure 2.

Figure 2. Costs of unintended pregnancy.

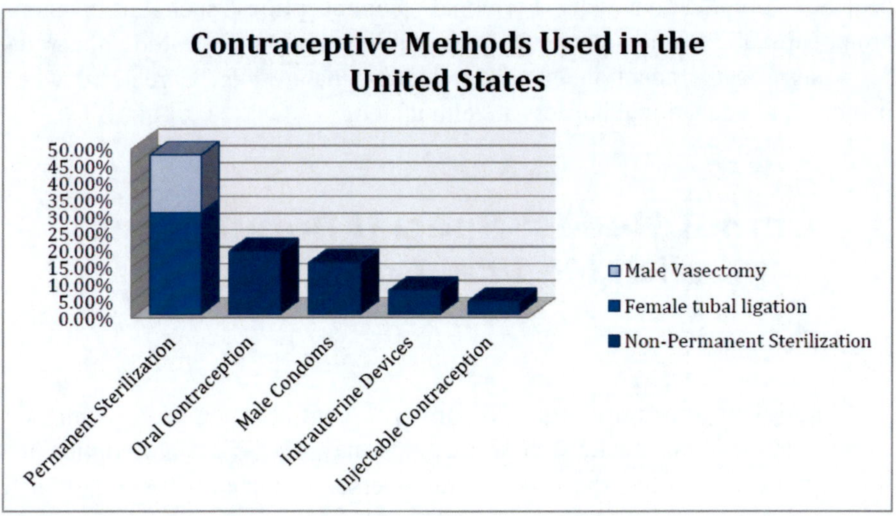

Figure 3. Contraceptive methods in the United States.

The safety, efficacy, availability and acceptability of each contraceptive method must be considered when choosing the most appropriate method. The effectiveness of a method is heavily dependent on the consistent and correct usage, both of which can vary greatly depending on the age, income, and culture of the user. Options such as the LARC methods provide highly effective contraception because they eliminate the need for daily or weekly compliance from the patient. However, there is still relatively low use likely due to misconceptions from both providers and patients.

The Contraceptive CHOICE Project was a landmark project that provided no cost contraception as well as patient and provider education in an effort to decrease unintended pregnancy. This cohort study was performed from 2007 to 2011 in the St. Louis, Missouri region and enrolled 9,250 women ages 14-45 years of age. Approximately 50% of the sample population consisted of minorities, many of whom were economically disadvantaged. Two-thirds of women chose a long-acting reversible contraception (LARC) method to include either an intrauterine device (37%) or an implant (34.5%) [27,28]. More importantly, 77% of women who chose a LARC method were still using it at 2 years compared to 41% who chose a non-long acting method[29]. Those women who chose a LARC method were also found to be 20 times less likely to have an unintended pregnancy in the first year [30]. The study was not designed to address the important issue of sexually transmitted infections or medical complications of hormonal contraception such as venous thromboembolism in this presumably healthy population. This study illustrates that a significant reduction in unintended pregnancy can be realized when financial and educational barriers are eliminated.

Unmet Needs: Special Populations with Medical Conditions

Overview

Historically, the most effective forms of contraception have contained hormones [31]. Unfortunately these methods may not be a viable option for women with medical conditions that are adversely affected by estradiol such as heart disease, diabetes with vascular involvement, gynecological cancers (endometrial or ovarian), epilepsy, sickle cell disease, stroke, thrombogenic mutations, and systemic lupus erythematous[4]. The development of estrogen free contraceptive methods such as Depo-Provera™ and the intrauterine devices has helped overcome some of these concerns, and decrease the unmet need in these women.

However, even with these viable options for the at risk patients, there are still a fair number of patients who are not using any methods. In addition, there are many women who are candidates for hormonal contraception who are denied access to these forms of birth control because their providers assume they have an absolute contraindication to hormonal contraception. Although there are a small number of women with medical conditions that contraindicate estrogen use (Figure 4), there are many more women with common conditions such as obesity, hypertension and smoking with a significant risk of complications who may use these methods with caution.

- Smoking and age 35 years or older
- Less than 21 days postpartum or 21–42 days postpartum with other risk factors
- Major surgery with prolonged immobilization
- History of deep vein thrombosis or pulmonary embolism
- Hereditary thrombophilia (including antiphospholipid syndrome)
- Inflammatory bowel disease with active or extensive disease, surgery, immobilization, corticosteroid use, vitamin deficiencies, or fluid depletion
- Systemic lupus erythematosus with positive (or unknown) antiphospholipid antibodies

*Oral contraceptive use in women with these conditions is classified as U.S. Medical Eligibility Criteria Category 3 (theoretical or proven risks usually outweigh the advantages of using the method) or Category 4 (condition that represents an unacceptable health risk if the contraceptive method is used).

Data from U.S. Medical Eligibility Criteria for Contraceptive Use, 2010. Centers for Disease Control and Prevention (CDC). MMWR Recomm Rep 2010;59(RR-4):1–86 and Update to CDC's U.S. Medical Eligibility Criteria for Contraceptive Use, 2010: revised recommendations for the use of contraceptive methods during the postpartum period. Centers for Disease Control and Prevention (CDC). MMWR Morb Mortal Wkly Rep 2011;60:878–83.

Source: Risk of venous thromboembolism among users of drospirenone-containing oral contraceptive pills. Committee Opinion No.540. American College of Obstetricians and Gynecologists. *Obstetrics and Gynecology.* 120,1239 (2012).

Figure 4. High-risk factors for venous thromboembolism in users of combined oral contraceptives.*

Venous Thromboembolism

It is well recognized there is an increased risk of venous thromboembolism with combined oral contraceptive (COC) use, particularly because of the estrogen component[32,33]and specific formulations that include the progestins desogestrel or gestodene[34,35]. Among all COC users, the risk of VTE is 3-9/10,000 women. This is slightly higher than the risk of non-contraceptive users who are not pregnant or taking hormones, estimated to be 1-5/10,000 women [36]. However, both risks are still low when compared to the risk of thromboembolism during a pregnancy, which is 5-20/10,000 women and during the postpartum period, 40-65/10,000 women [36]. Thus, the benefit of COCs, even taking into account the associated risk of VTE, may still outweigh the significant higher risk of VTE during pregnancy and in the postpartum period (Figure 5) [37].

Due to this known increased risk of VTE with COC, research has been dedicated to finding other contraceptive options for these particular high-risk patients. Methods such as progesterone only pills and intrauterine devices have been found to have no association with venous thrombosis [32,38], thus making them viable options.

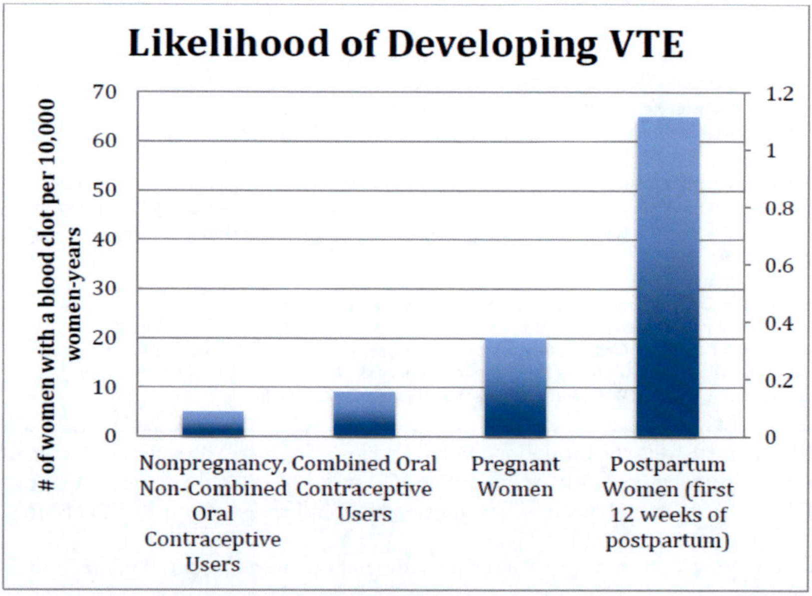

Figure generated with data from: Food and Drug Administration. FDA drug safety communication: updated information about the risk of blood clots in women taking birth control pills containing drospirenone. Silver Spring (MD): FDA; 2012. Available at: http://www.fda.gov/Drugs/ DrugSafety/ucm299305. Accessed September 10, 2014.

Figure 5. Likelihood of developing blood clot, maximum range.

Obesity

Obesity remains a leading public health concern in the American population [39,40] and plays a significant role in increasing the risk of VTE with combined oral contraceptive users [41-43]. Currently, more than one-third of adult U.S. women are obese (defined as BMI greater than 30), of which 8% are in the extreme obese category (defined as BMI greater than 40) [44]. Obesity has been shown to be associated with an increase in pro-coagulant factors such as factor VII, factor VIII, factor XII, and fibrinogen [45]. These factors cause a pro-coagulant effect and hence, hypercoagulability. Thus, at a baseline, obese patients are at an increased risk of venous thrombosis [42,45,46]. One study reported a 2.4 fold increased risk of VTE among obese women than their normal weight female counterpart [42]. Furthermore, obese women who use combined oral contraception are found to have a upwards of a 10-fold increase in VTE risk [42]. This highlights the importance of providing obese women with safer contraceptive options.

Another concern for obese women using contraception is the potential change in the absorption and the volume of distribution of combined oral contraceptive pills when compared to thinner patients [47]. Recent studies evaluating the effectiveness of hormonal contraception with increased BMI have been controversial. For example, Zieman and colleagues demonstrated decreased effectiveness of the combined contraceptive patch in women weighing > 90 kg [48]. Along the same lines, Holt and colleagues performed a retrospective cohort analysis in overweight women (BMI >25) looking primarily at the oral form of combined hormonal contraception and demonstrated similar results [49]. Obese women may have greater hypothalamic-pituitary-ovarian axis activity even on COC when compared to normal weight women, possibly leading to unwanted ovulation and unplanned pregnancy [50]. However, others have indicated no difference in efficacy of oral contraception with an increased BMI [51,52]. This debate illustrates the need for further research and studies to develop safer, efficacious, estrogen free contraception in the growing overweight and obese population.

Tobacco Use, Vascular, and Cardiovascular Disease

Tobacco smokers using first or second generation COC are at a higher risk for cardiovascular disease, especially myocardial infarctions [53]. They are also at an increased risk of stroke and peripheral artery disease [54,55].

Accordingly, the Centers for Disease Control and Prevention (CDC) recommends any women smokers over the age of 35 who smoke more than 15 cigarettes per day should not use COCs[4]. The lack of use of COCs by this population, however, exposes them to the significant risk of thromboembolic complications that accompany an unplanned pregnancy [36,37].

Inherited and Acquired Thrombophilias

The risk of venous thromboembolism increases substantially with inherited thrombophilias among COC users. Common inherited thrombophilias include Factor V Leiden, Prothrombin G20210A, Protein C Deficiency, Protein S Deficiency, and Antithrombin Deficiency. The most prevalent disorder among these is Factor V Leiden heterozygous, affecting approximately 1-15% of the general population [56]. For Factor V Leiden homozygous women who are not using oral contraceptives, the risk of thrombosis rises 8-fold. For those who are using oral contraceptives, the risk increases to more than 30-fold (Figure 6) [57]. This highlights the importance of choosing a safe, but still highly effective form of birth control for women of the reproductive age with Factor V Leiden who wish to have some sort of contraception.

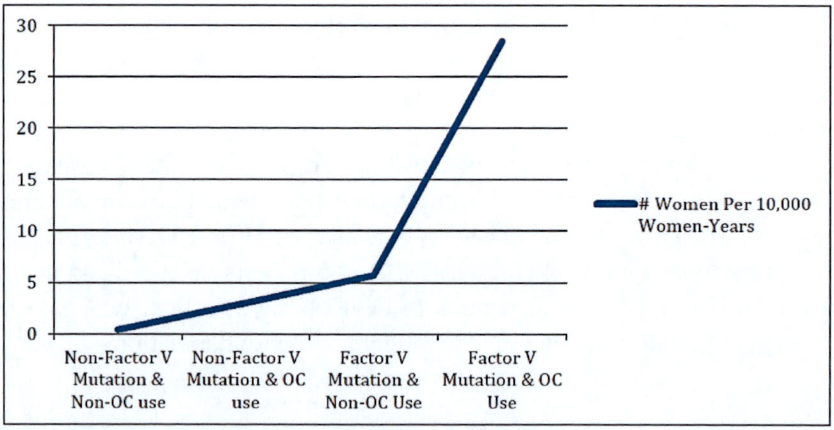

Figure generated from data from: Vandenbroucke JP, van der Meer FJ, Helmerhorst FM, Rosendaal FR. *Bmj*. 313,1127 (1996).

Figure 6. Risks of thrombosis associated with Factor V Leiden mutation and oral contraceptive (OC) use.

Along the same argument, acquired thrombophilias encompass conditions that can increase the risk of thrombosis. Examples would include antiphospholipid syndrome, sickle cell disease, myeloproliferative disorders, and cancers. At this time, the best non-barrier choices for patients with inherited and acquired thrombophilias include progesterone-only options like the levonorgestrel intrauterine device, progestin-only pills and Depo-Provera.

Systemic Lupus Erythematous

Providers are often reluctantto prescribe oral contraceptives to patients with Systemic Lupus Erythematous (SLE). One main concern is the potential for exogenous hormones to contribute to lupus flares [58]. Despite these concerns, reproductive aged women with SLE should have access to safe and effective birth control [59]. This was the primary question of the Oral Contraceptive-Safety of Estrogens in Lupus Erythematosus National Assessment Trial (OC-SELENA). This randomized, placebo-controlled multicenter study demonstrated oral contraceptives were not associated with an increase in severe, mild-moderate, or total flares over a one-year period. The investigators concluded that combined oral contraceptive pills containing estrogen is a valid birth-control option for patients with inactive or stable, moderate SLE who are low risk for thrombosis [60,61]. Increased education among providers and patients may help decrease the reluctance to provide a safe form of birth control to this population.

Neurologic Disorders

Common neurologic disorders such as migraine headaches, limit the types of contraceptives that can be offered. Migraines are the most common type of headaches in young adults, experienced by almost 25% of all women by their mid to late 30s [62]. In combined oral contraceptive users, the risk of an ischemic stroke was twice as likely in women who had a history of migraines compared to those with no history of migraines [63,64]. The importance of offering adequate contraception that does not raise the risk of adverse events remains a public health concern given that migraines and oral contraception are both independent risk factors for strokes [38,65].

Additionally, 41 women in 100,000 person years in the United States are diagnosed with seizures or epilepsy [66]. Antiepileptic medication use is relatively common in reproductive age women and its use impacts the efficacy of oral contraceptives. One trial demonstrated an increase in seizure activity when using both COCS and Lamotrigine [67]. This population needs a contraceptive method that does not decrease the epilepsy threshold[68]. Among this group of patients, there seems to exist a significant gap of knowledge regarding this interaction, especially among teenagers. An online survey and 12 online focus group discussions performed from 2012 to 2013 polled female teenagers with epilepsy. All the participants desired increased guidance from providers to help support their contraceptive decisions[69] illustrating not only the need for additional methods that will benefit medically, but also the need to increase counseling and knowledge in this unmet needs group.

Human Immunodeficiency Virus

In the U.S., thousands of reproductive aged women who are living with HIV have a need for effective contraception that is not impacted by their antiretroviral (ARV) medication. Antiretroviral therapy drugs have the potential to change the bioavailability of the steroid hormones in hormonal contraceptives [70]. Though there is only limited data, evidence suggests interactions that may alter the safety and effectiveness of both ARV therapy and COC [71]. For instance, if an HIV positive woman taking protease inhibitors, such as Darunavir, Fos/amprenavir, Lopinavir, Saquinavir, or Tipranavir, is started on COC, it is strongly recommended to also use condoms consistently to prevent HIV transmission and to compensate for any possible decrease in effectiveness of the COC[72-74]. On the other hand, ARV options like Tenofovir or Maraviroc have been shown to have no effect on effectiveness of COC [74-76]. At this time, contraception options exclusive of barrier methods such as male or female condoms do not protect again HIV. The challenge is to develop better options that are not affected by ARV therapy, in addition to decreasing transmission rates of HIV from partner to partner.

Though there have been a number of studies that have focused on adult women with HIV, few studies have looked at adolescents and young adults, a group that represents 40% of the HIV population. Robinson and colleagues interviewed 10 HIV positive women ages 13-21 years [77]. Of significance, these participants identified their HIV care provider as their primary source of information regarding contraception. This underscores the unmet needs for family planning services and the importance of collaboration among HIV care providers and adolescent-friendly family planning providers.

Unmet Needs: Special Population

Economically Disadvantaged

A major concern for reproductive aged women with low incomes is the substantial cost of contraception, leading to increased use of more cost-effective traditional methods. This includes withdrawal or interval abstinence, which is shown to be less effective at preventing pregnancies [78]. These women are also more likely to have unprotected intercourse in the context of financial difficulties with continued sexual activity [79]. Between the years of 1994 and 2001, Finer and colleagues found women in the lowest income bracket had much higher unintended pregnancy rates compared to wealthier women [21]. Specifically, the unintended pregnancy rate among women below the poverty line was 112 per 1,000 women. Comparatively, women with incomes twice the poverty level had much lower pregnancy rates, close to 29 per 1,000 women. Thus, the unintended pregnancies among those with lower income were almost four times higher than their more financially stable counterparts (Figure 7) [21].

In identifying the most cost-effective contraceptive option, it is important to consider efficacy as well as finances. The most affordable long-term methods, while having the best effectiveness, are the copper T-IUD, the levonorgestrel IUD, and a vasectomy [52,80-82]. Though an IUD requires a larger upfront cost of $500 to $1,000, the cost averaged over the device's lifespan of 5-10 years is approximately $100 per year. As a comparison, condoms can average $3 each. For a couple that uses them twice a week, the cost can rise to $250 per year, $150 more than the annual cost of an IUD. For a male patient, vasectomies can cost between $350 and $1,000. Averaged over 20 years, the annual cost can be as low as $30[52]. Thus, vasectomies may be the most cost-effective method over the long-term for low-income families but requires more education to increase its cultural acceptability (Figure 8).

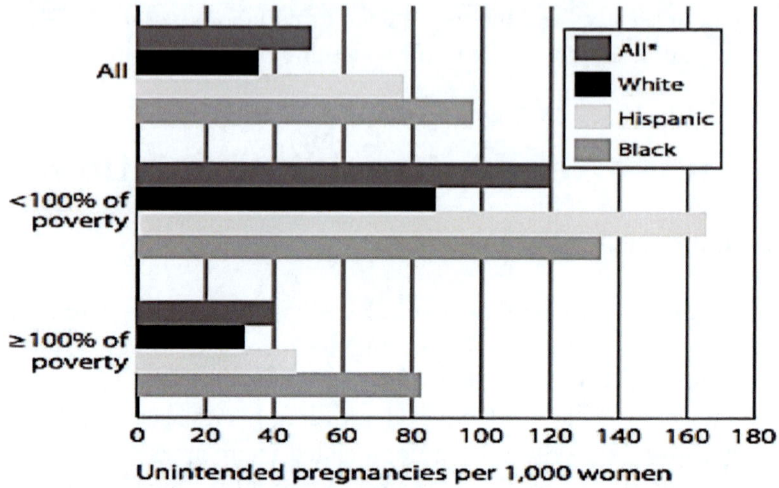

Source: Finer LB and Henshaw SK, Disparities in rates of unintended pregnancy in the United States, 1994 and 2001, Perspectives on Sexual and Reproductive Health, 2006, 38(2):90–96, Figure 2.

Figure 7. Unintended pregnancy rate by race, ethnicity, and income. *Excludes women who are not white, Hispanic, or black.

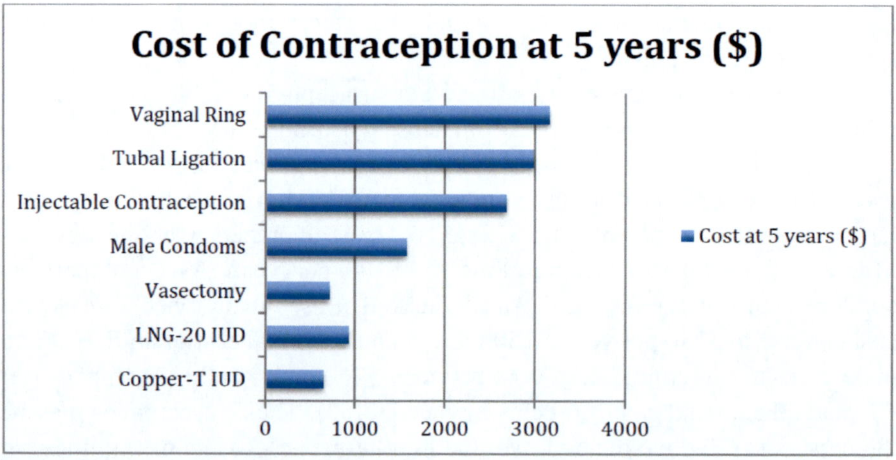

Figure generated from data from: Trussell J, Lalla AM, Doan QV, Reyes E, Pinto L, Gricar J. *Contraception*. 79,5 (2009).

Figure 8. Cost of contraception at 5 years. The Copper T-IUD, LNG-20 IUD, and vasectomy have the lowest cost over a 5-year period. LNG-20 IUD: Levonorgestrel-20 intrauterine device.

In 2010, Congress enacted the Affordable Care Act (ACA) that advocates the idea that healthcare is a right, not a privilege [83]. The ACA had a goal of lowering the cost of healthcare and reducing the number of uninsured individuals who presumably did not have access to care. Prior to the implementation of the ACA, nineteen million women ages 18-64 years were uninsured [84]. In 2009, it was estimated 25% of all uninsured Americans chose not to use preventative medical care because of cost [85] compared to only 4% of privately insured adults [86]. Under this Act, preventative services such as contraception are covered in addition to excluding cost sharing; both designed to help women overcome financial barriers to contraception. It has been shown that even small amounts of cost sharing decreases the use of preventative health care like contraception, especially among low-income Americans [87]. This law helps make health care more accessible and more affordable to millions of Americans (Figure 9).

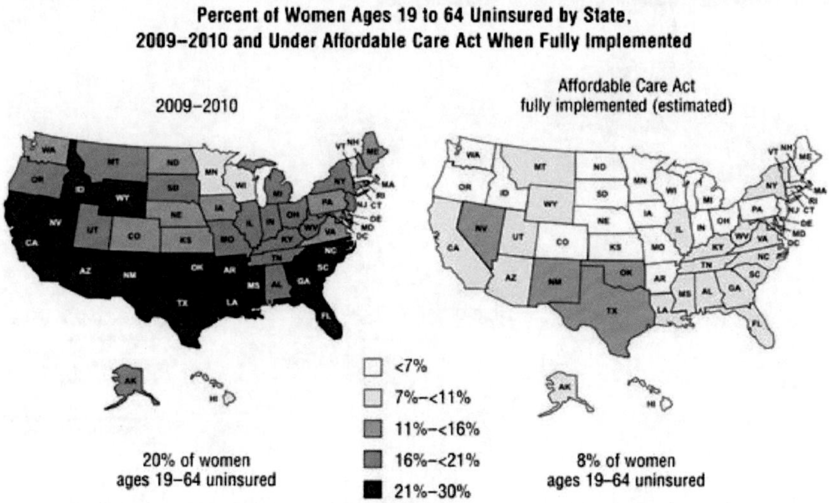

Source: R Robertson, D Squires, T. Garber, S.R. Collins, and M.M. Doty. Realizing Health Reform's Potential. Oceans Apart: The Higher Health Costs of Women in the U.S. Compared to Other Nations, and How Reform Is Helping, The Commonwealth Fund, 2012.

Figure 9. Percent of women ages 19 to 64 uninsured by state, 2009-2010 and under the Affordable Care Act when fully implemented.

As a means to further improve access to care, the Supreme Court ruled in 2012 that states could expand their Medicaid programs by basing eligibility just on income. The states who choose to opt out of this program cannot be punished with the withdrawal of federal Medicaid funds (Figure 10), however can be denied additional federal funds for Medicaid. If all states participated in this Medicaid expansion, it is estimated that the number of uninsured women, aged 19-64, will be reduced from 20% to 8% [88].

As the number of uninsured women decreases, the number of contraceptive users increases. From the Fall of 2012 to the Spring of 2013, there was a significant increase in the proportion of privately insured oral contraceptive users and vaginal ring users. The proportion of women paying nothing out of pocket among the pill users increased from 15% to 40% while vaginal ring users increased from 23% to 52% [89]. The ACA will hopefully continue to result in increased access to contraception, and consequently a decrease in unintended pregnancy rates.

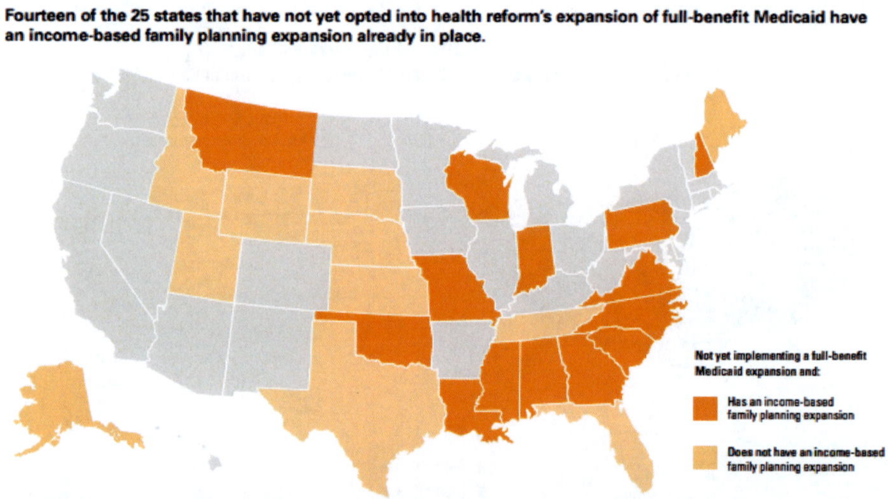

Source: Sonfield A, Hasstedt K and Gold RB, Moving Forward: Family Planning in the Era of Health Reform, New York: Guttmacher Institute, 2014, Figure 4.5, p. 30.

Figure 10. States that have not yet opted into health reform's expansion of full-benefit Medicaid have an income-based family planning expansion already in place.

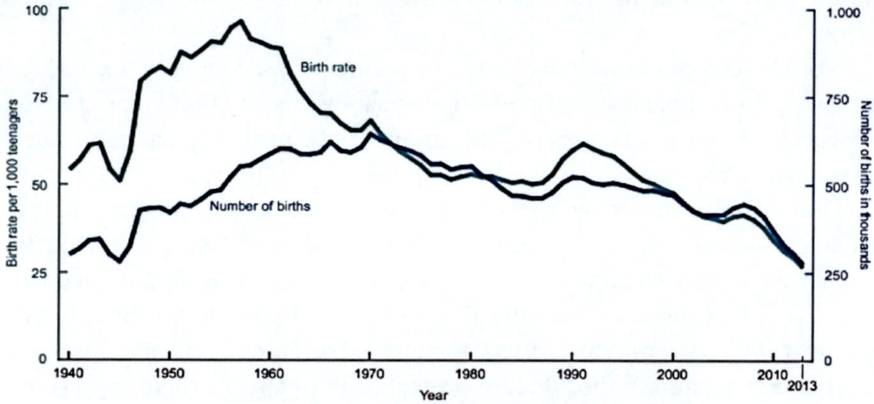

Source: Ventura SJ, Hamilton BE, Matthews TJ. National and state patterns of teen births in the United States, 1940-2013. National vital statistics reports : vol 63 no 4. Hyattsville, MD: National Center for Health Statistics. 2014.

Figure 11. Number of births and birth rates for teenagers aged 15-19: United States, 1940-2013.

Adolescents

Teen pregnancies in the United States have declined since its peak in 1957 (Figure 11). With the exception of short periods of time where rates increased slightly, there has been a steady decline in birth rates that can be generalized among all race, ethnicity groups, and states [90,91]. In 2013, the birth rate was 26.6 births per 1,000 teenagers between the ages of 15-19 years, which was less than one-half of the birth rate in 1991 of 61.8 per 1,000 teenagers. This ultimately translates to 4 million fewer teenage births from 1992 to 2012[92].

Despite a decrease in pregnancy rates, the number of sexually active teenagers has not decreased dramatically [93]; thus the downward trend of birth rates is likely due to the increased contraceptive use by teenagers in the past several years [94]. It is known that sexual activity is rare among those younger than 12 years, however increases to 30% between the ages of 15-17. By the age of 17 years, 40% of adolescents are sexually active. By the age of 19 years, almost 70% have had intercourse (Figure 12) [21]. Among all teenagers, girls who are 14 years or younger are less likely to have used a method of Contraception at first sex and will take longer to begin using contraception [95]. Comparatively, 78% of sexually active older female teens and 85% of their male counterparts reported using contraceptive methods during their first sexual experience [96].

The choice of contraception for adolescents is based on easy access, easy use, and low financial cost. Male condoms meet these criteria and consequently, there was a rise of use from 42.6% to 62.8% among sexually active high school students from 1991 to 2007 (Figure 13) [97].

Despite this, consistent use of any method of contraception remains a challenge among this age group. The option of long-acting contraceptive methods provides a solution to this problem. However, the upfront high cost of an IUD and reticence to placing an IUD in a nulliparous adolescent female by providers [98] present real barriers for teenagers. Over a seven year period, with better education to health care providers and patients, there has been an increase in LARC methods from 0.3% use among teenagers in 2002 to 4.5% in 2009[99]. As illustrated in the CHOICE project where financial barriers were removed and education was provided, 50% of women between 18 and 20 years of age chose an intrauterine device as their contraception and 40% of those between 14 and 17 years of age chose the long acting implant [30]. Importantly, these young women had higher satisfaction, better continuation of these methods, in addition to being 20 times less likely to have an unintended pregnancy than those who chose a short-term method like the COC or the patch [30].

Because of compliance issues among adolescents, long-acting reversible contraception methods, to include intrauterine devices and implants, offer an excellent choice for this group. It has also been proven to be one of the most effective methods in decreasing the rate of unintended pregnancies in adolescents [100]. However, the issue of the significant financial cost needs to be addressed. For an adolescent, there are several options to approach this financial barrier, however none are ideal. This includes using a parent's insurance which notifies the parent of the child's choice, utilizing government funded programs such as Medicaid or a Title X family planning clinic which adolescents may not be fully aware of, or paying out-of pocket at cost-prohibitive rates.

Most commonly, adolescents receive services through their state's family planning clinics. In 2006, 25% of nearly two million women who received care at a planning center were under the age of 20[88]. An impressive state model is the Colorado Family Planning Initiative, which offered low-income women free or low-cost LARC methods. It was supported by a $23 million anonymous donation and provided more than 30,000 IUDs or implants given by the state's 68 family planning clinics. From the years 2009 to 2013, there was a 40% decline in teen birth rates [101] dramatically decreasing the state's teen birth rate. Using Colorado as a state model, easier access and more affordable options may help increase the usage of this highly effective contraceptive method.

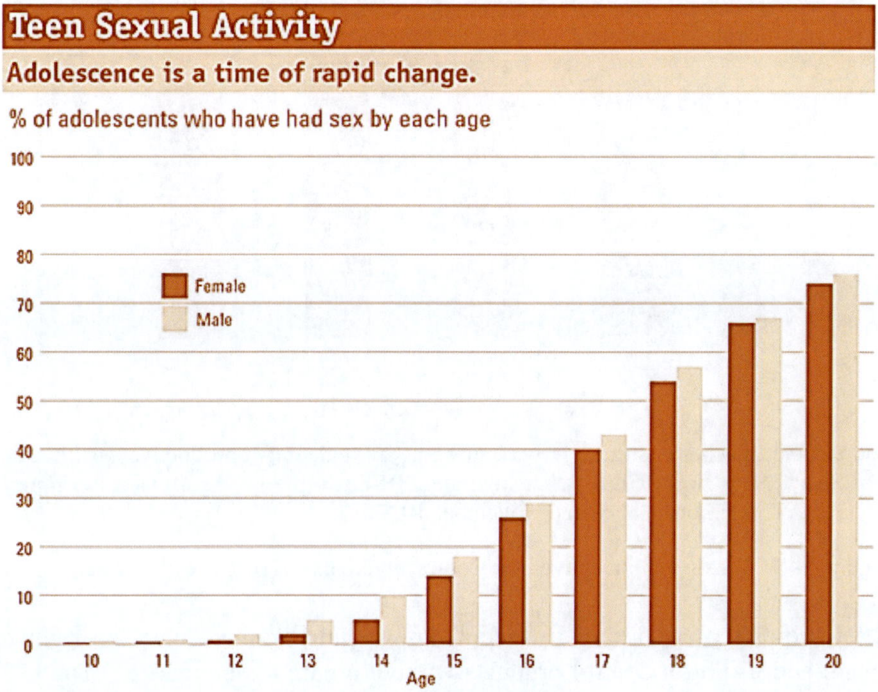

Source: Guttmacher Institute, American teens' sexual and reproductive health, fact sheet, New York: Guttmacher Institute, 2014, <http://www.guttmacher.org/ pubs/ FB-ATSRH.html>, accessed November 10, 2014.

Figure 12. Teen Sexual Activity.

On a social level, it has been shown that open communication between adolescents and parents about sex and birth control leads to an increased use of condoms and other contraceptive use [102]. Up to 80% of teenagers stated it would be easier to avoid teen pregnancies if they were able to have more open, honest conversations with their parents. There were 63% of adolescents that reported the primary reason they do not use contraception is because they are afraid their parents will find out [103]. Clear communication between parents and children is important and may alter sexual decision making during their teenage years [104].

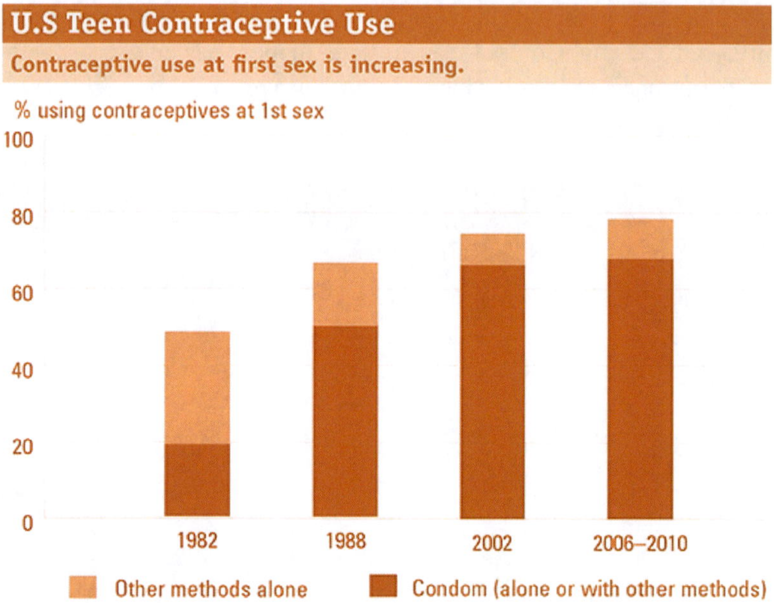

Source: Guttmacher Institute, American teens' sexual and reproductive health, Fact Sheet, New York: Guttmacher Institute, 2014, <http://www.guttmacher.org/pubs/FB-ATSRH.html>, accessed November 10, 2014.

Figure 13. U.S. teen contraceptive use. Contraceptive use at first sex is increasing.

Importantly, according to federal law, young women have the right to obtain and use birth control products without a parent's permission. The U.S. Supreme Court ruled the constitutional right to privacy extends to a minor's decision to access and use contraception. This ruling highlighted that although parental involvement was desirable, it is not mandatory [105]. Specifically, the Title X and Medicaid programs do not require parental consent [106]. However, regulations on parents' consent with private insurance vary from state to state. Currently, 26 states and the District of Columbia allow teens, 12 years and older, to seek family planning options without parental consent; 20 states allow only in certain situations; and 4 states have no policy regarding this issue [107]. Per the Center for Reproductive Rights, if minors were required to tell a parent before they could access contraception, teenagers would delay or would simply not seek services, but would not reduce sexual activity [106]. Among this special population, there is a need for discrete, easily administered contraception. The key to success is having a keen sensitivity to the adolescents need to have their privacy respected.

The topic of education regarding the sexual behavior of adolescents has long been the subject of debate for the past couple centuries in the U.S and seemingly always resulting in a deadlock. On one side, advocates of a comprehensive sex education emphasize the importance of both abstinence and contraception counseling, in addition to discussions about healthy relationships, parent-child communication, and decision-making skills. On the other side of the debate, advocates champion abstinence education among teenagers, teaching points such as a faithful monogamous relationship in the context of a marriage should be the only context for human sexual activity [85]. In the past several years, Congress has shifted their support from abstinence only teaching to prevention efforts that focus more on comprehensive education [108]. From 2011 to 2014, new teenage pregnancy prevention programs have been funded by more than $100 million in support of this new idea [85].

Racial, Cultural, and Ethnic Issues

There are differences in the choice of contraceptive use and the number of users among different racial populations in the United States. Per the U.S. Department of Health and Human Services, 66% of non-Hispanic white women were using a form of contraception compared with 60% of Hispanic women and 54% of non-Hispanic black women. From 2006-2010, the most common contraceptive methods were female sterilization and the oral contraceptive pill (Figure 14). 32% of white women chose to use the pill, compared to 21% of Asians, 17-23% of Hispanics, and 18% of African American women. Conversely, 37% of African American women and foreign-born Hispanic women were more likely to use female sterilization compared to 24% of white women, 27% of U.S.-born Hispanic women, and 11% of Asian women. The use of barrier methods like condoms were highest among Asian women at 40% compared to the overall average of 16% of condom usage among other racial groups. The use of LARCs, specifically IUDs is on the rise across all racial groups [26] likely because of better education and easier access to care. Still, even with greater than 50% usage of some form of contraceptive method among all racial groups, the number of women *not* using any form of contraception is significant.

The number of unintended pregnancy rates among these different racial groups illustrates the need for continued push to improve contraception usage. Within the first year of using a new contraceptive method, 10% of non-

Hispanic white women will have an unintended pregnancy. This increases to 15% for Hispanic women and up to 20% for non-Hispanic black women [26]. These unintended pregnancy rates among these groups did not alter significantly from 2001 to 2006[21] demonstrating the need for targeted interventions to address proper usage of contraception among all groups.

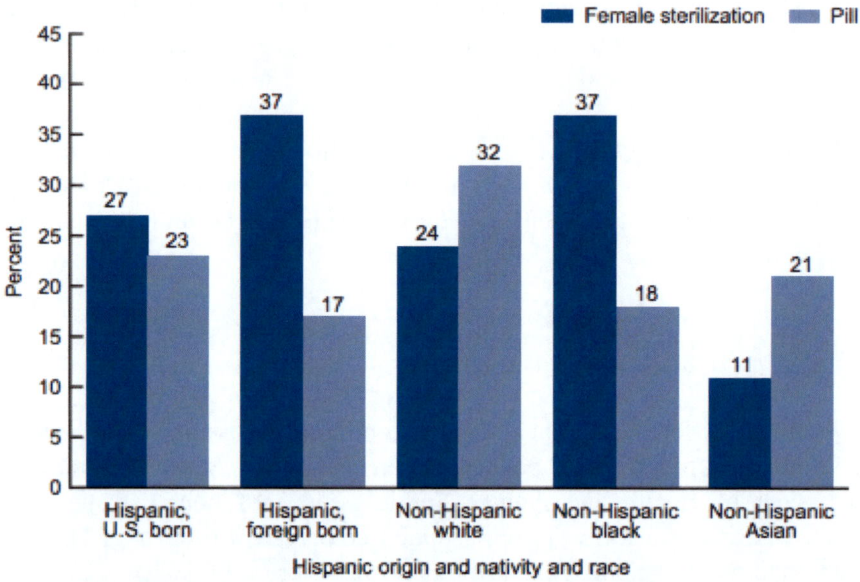

Source: Jones J, Mosher W, Daniels K. Current contraceptive use in the United States, 2006-2010, and changes in patterns of use since 1995. National health statistics reports; no 60. Hyattsville, MD: National Center for Health Statistics. 2012.

Figure 14. Percentage of women using female sterilization and the pill compared between difference racial groups in the United States from 2006-2010.

Religious beliefs are widely assumed to have an impact on contraceptive use, with positions varying among different groups. For many women, religion plays a significant role in influencing decisions about birth control. The highest rates of unintended pregnancy were among women with no religious affiliations, followed by Catholics, and then Protestants [21]. Historically, the Roman Catholic Church has remained firm on its position prohibiting artificial contraception with the idea that a new life starts at the moment of conception [109]. Within Catholicism, the main purpose of marriage and sexual intercourse is procreation, thus contraception inhibits and violates this purpose [110]. Abstinence and the rhythm method are the only officially approved methods, with all other forms, including emergency contraception, viewed as a sin [111]. It was not until 1930, when the non-Catholic Christians, specifically the Anglican Communion, changed the policy on accepting modern contraception. Soon after, Protestant groups also came to accept the use of modern contraception [112]. Currently, most liberal Christian communities now assent to the use of contraception within a marriage, leaving the decision of which method to use up to the discretion of the couple [113].

Similarly, the opinion on contraception in the Islamic culture varies widely, with some arguing that it should be prohibited and others stating it is allowed but discouraged [114,115]. Fundamentalist Muslims affirm that any form of contraception violates God's intent [116]; however the majority of Muslims permit modern methods as long as they are reversible, do not cause abortion, and are used only within marriage [115-117]. The prevalence of contraceptive use among Muslim women in the United States varies substantially depending on personal and family beliefs [118]. The patient's family country of origin may play an integral part on the level of acceptance of contraception. The prevalence of contraceptive use in different Muslin countries varies widely from less than 5% countries like Sudan, Somalia, and Mauritania to more than 50% in others such as Turkey and Lebanon[119], demonstrating the wide range of approval. For Muslim women, there are traditional pressures to include familial and religious influences that affect the decision to procreate [120]. In addition, other factors that hinder contraceptive use include misconceptions about side effects of modern methods, the association of fertility with femininity, and the low status of women in certain communities [115,120,121].

Within the Orthodox Judaism community, birth control is generally not encouraged [122]. However, when it is used, husbands need to be informed of, and approve of, the use [123,124]. Traditional contraceptive methods of abstinence and the rhythm method are not acceptable in addition to any male sterilization techniques that would impair the male reproductive organs [110,125]. The most acceptable form of contraception is oral contraceptives, but also diaphragms and spermicide. Intra-uterine devices are controversial since if implantation of a fertilized ovum is prevented, it may be looked at as a form of abortion [110,125] though no evidence exists to support this. Though religion weighs heavily on a couples decision, the ultimate choice of contraception is largely influenced by other factors such as the intended fertility control needs, peer influence, the number of current children, the age of the women, and the education of the couple [126].

In sharp contrast to a number of religions, Hinduism regards all contraceptive methods as acceptable[127,128], believing that it is a personal matter for women and the choice of usage is not within the scope of religious injunction. However, despite religious permissibility, there prevails a lack of family planning among Hindu women[121]. Factors that can explain this are cultural resistance, sexism, lack of female empowerment and decreased accessibility to services [121,129].

There is a clear importance of religion in making decisions about contraceptive use. However, even with the prohibition of modern contraception in certain religions, studies have shown that 95% of women in North America have used some form of contraceptive method at some point in their lives [130]. Health care providers must be aware of religious, social and cultural views when counseling on contraception. Perhaps more importantly, providers should remember that each woman is individual and her personal views on contraception may not mirror those of her religious teachings.

Unmet Contraceptive Needs of Women at Risk of High Mortality Viruses

There is a global need for contraception among reproductive aged women who may be exposed to viruses that carry increased maternal morbidity and mortality. One such high-risk virus among the general population is the H1N1 or Influenza A virus, which reached a global pandemic in 2009. Pregnant women affected with the H1N1 virus are at a substantially higher risk of hospitalization compared to the general population, in addition to accounting for 5% of deaths caused by the influenza virus[131].Fortunately, the development of the influenza vaccination has been shown to reduce the risk of illness to the patient and her infant during the first 6 months of life [132].In addition, there are decreased adverse outcomes for infants whose mother received the vaccine, such as small size for gestational age and preterm birth[131]. Though there are now improved antiviral therapies and the availability of a vaccination, preventing undesired pregnancies with its associated increased risks among reproductive aged women may help decrease the overall morbidity and mortality associated with the H1N1 virus.

More recently in 2014, the largest outbreak of the Ebola virus was seen affecting thousands of people in West Africa including reproductive aged women, pregnant women, and neonates. After months of rapid spread of the

Ebola Virus, the World Health Organization declared a Public Health Emergency of International Concern [133-134] currently; there is limited data about sexual transmission of the Ebola virus, the effects on pregnancy, and horizontal transmission to the fetus. However, what has been reported is alarming with maternal morbidity exceeding 95% in those affected with hemorrhagic fever [135].There is also evidence of increased risk of spontaneous abortion and pregnancy-associated hemorrhage [136]. Similarly, it has been reported that fetal and newborn mortality comes close to 100% when affected by the virus [137] which is also transmittable through breast milk, thus contraindicating breast-feeding. It should also be noted that deliveries are high-risk situations for exposure for uninfected healthcare personnel as are all surgical interventions.

The importance of contraception in reproductive age women should be emphasized for those are at risk for exposure to the Ebola virus. The virus can be transmitted through direct contact of skin or mucous membranes with blood or body fluids, in addition to sexual transmission as semen carries the virus for up to 7 weeks after recovery from the infection[138-139].Per the United States Army Medical Research Institute of Infectious Disease, a period of 3 months is recommended to avoid sexual contact to decrease contraction rates[140] .Ensuring easy access to contraception, particularly condoms, should be considered a crucial preventative strategy to decrease sexual transmission of the Ebola Virus and the potential subsequent pregnancy consequences.

As of 2014, efforts are ongoing to develop safe and effective vaccinations against Ebola virus, which have proven to be the key to eradicating similar viral outbreaks. Given the high mortality to mothers and babies when infected, in cases where the likelihood of infection is high, contraception should also be offered as standard of care. In the case of high-mortality viruses for which vaccinations and other therapies exist, a contraception plan should concurrently be implemented given that the disease course is so much more lethal in the context of pregnancy.

Addressing Unmet Contraceptive Needs

Since the 1970s, there has been increasing global awareness about the importance of addressing unmet contraceptive needs. Organizations such as the American College of Obstetricians and Gynecologists have published potential ways to help improve contraceptive access and use. One suggested strategy is to make oral contraceptives available over-the counter with self-screening for contraindications using pre-set checklists [3]. In a 2004 national telephone survey of 811 women in the reproductive years, 68% of women stated they would utilize pharmacy access for contraception if it were available. Perhaps more importantly, 46% of uninsured women and 40% of low-income women who were not using contraception at the time of the survey stated they would start using COCs if it were more accessible [141]. Similarly, a national survey of 2,725 pharmacists showed 85% would be interested in providing hormonal contraception [142]. As a part of the Contraceptive CHOICE Project, a chart review was completed that showed only 24 of 1,010 participants who desired a combined hormonal contraception had a true medical contraindication to its use [143].This low prevalence of women with true contraindications supports the idea of over-the-counter contraception with self-screening.

Along with easier access to contraception, there are ongoing efforts to provide for better contraceptive options. New technologies to improve different contraception types have been the focus of many researchers in the past couple decades. In order to help decrease the number of adverse events associated with the estrogen component of COCs, different formulations of reduced dosage of estrogen have been used [144] New progestogens have been studied such as dienogest, nomegestrol, and drospirenone in COCs to help decrease undesirable side effects [145,146] .The development of efficacious estrogen-free oral contraception is another step towards an acceptable and safer option of those with medical contraindications to estrogen.

Intrauterine devices have emerged as a safe and effective long-term contraception for the majority of women. Unfortunately, it may not be chosen due to provider discomfort with the insertion, patient fear of painful placement, or patient and providers' lack of education. To counter the first two problems, there have been different proposed designs of IUDs which have a simple push-in technique with less pain during insertion in nulliparous women [147]. There are experimental versions of IUDs, which are "frameless" to decrease the pain during insertion [148] .Initial studies show good clinical results, however there is a need for more published data on efficacy prior to release to the public. To counter the latter issue, additional education should target providers with subsequent improved counseling to patients about LARC methods.

The idea of a reversible male contraception has been the focus of research for many years but none have been approved to date. It is known that many men are willing to take on adverse side effects and any possible health risks associated with contraceptive use[149] .Parallel to this, women have stated that they would welcome the availability of a reversible male contraception and would trust their partners to take it[150]. Progress in this field has been slow partly due to difficulties in finding an appropriate testosterone formulation to fully suppress sperm effectively[144] .The most promising regimens have been testosterone with an oral or implantable progesterone, however none have resulted in more than 95% azospermia[151]. The slow progress has also been largely due to lack of funding and low number of subjects in trials [144]. Regardless, if a male reversible contraception is developed, this has the potential of substantially influencing the unmet needs of women globally.

Conclusion

Though there has been substantial forward movement in addressing unmet contraceptive needs, there needs to be continued effort. The challenge is to provide care to all groups by focusing on specific populations as detailed above. The most common barriers to contraception that needs to be addressed are financial costs, access to care, lack of education on both provider and patient levels, better contraceptive method choice with certain medical conditions, and accounting for religious and cultural views.

An improvement in the education of LARC methods could likely be instrumental in both the increased use and the decrease in unintended pregnancies [152,153]. Illustrated by the Contraceptive CHOICE Project, once financial barriers were removed and education was provided, the majority of women chose a LARC method for contraception. [29]. The American Congress of Obstetricians and Gynecologists suggest LARC should be offered to all adolescents [100]. Colorado adapted these recommendations and implemented a program where LARC methods were offered for free or at a low-cost to low-income women. This change resulted in a dramatic decrease in teen birth rates in Colorado State illustrating how a change in state programs can significantly eliminate barriers for these young women [92]. This should serve as a model to all other states without similar programs. Programs such as this should encourage the implementation of comparable efforts to help decrease the unmet need for our youth. Greater LARC use and continuation can ultimately help reduce unintended pregnancies [154].

There is also a need for better dissemination of accurate contraceptive information especially among adolescents [155]. In addition, open communication about contraception between teenagers and parents has been shown to increase the use of contraception [102]. In this way, teens with access to their parent's private insurance may feel free to use it in acquiring contraceptive options. Other logistical barriers for teenagers and the financially disadvantaged include inaccessible locations, lack of transportation, and inconvenient clinic operating times. Better planning and awareness to have clinics built close to public transportation and more flexible hours may help with this issue [156].

In the past several years, there have been dramatic changes in the availability of contraception as the result of increasing government support related to the ACA. However, even as recently as June 2014, access to contraception has been impacted by legal challenges. In the recent ruling of the Burwell versus Hobby Lobby case, the court ruled that the ACA violated the Religious Freedom Restoration Act, a law passed by Congress in 1993 to ensure government would not interfere with a person's free exercise of religion. Hobby Lobby was granted an exemption from executing the ACA mandate with regards to contraceptive methods they felt could cause abortion such as the IUD or Plan B (emergency contraception). A compromise is being sought to provide emergency contraception (EC), and IUDs to women whose employers are granted religious exemption from providing them.

There is a continued need for a forward push to come up with new technologies for patients who cannot tolerate or are medically contraindicated to use current contraceptive methods. More funding and support is needed from the government level. However, improvements in current methods of contraception and also new future developments such as a male reversible contraception have the potential to dramatically alter the unmet need for women. Problems remain on the patient level, the provider level [152], and the healthcare system level. The challenge for everyone is to provide more affordable, more accessible, and more effective contraception to those who need it.

Unintended pregnancy is a multifactorial problem, which will require multiple solutions. Strategies directed at decreasing the unintended pregnancy rate must include greater contraceptive choices, improved access, better patient and provider education, and legislation and policies that will support these strategies. Tackling these specific issues addressed in this chapter allows us to be one step closer to meeting the unmet needs of reproductive aged women in the United States.

References

[1] Alkema, L; Kantorova, V; Menozzi, C; Biddlecom, A. *Lancet*. 381, 1642, (2013)

[2] United Nations. The Millennium Development Goals Report. 2011. http://www.un.org/millenniumgoals/pdf/ (2011_E) MDG Report 2011_Book LR.pdf, accessed August 20, 2014.

[3] *Obstetrics and gynecology*. 120,1527, (2012)

[4] Centers for Disease C, Prevention. U.S. Medical Eligibility Criteria for Contraceptive Use, 2010. Adapted from the World Health Organization Medical Eligibility Criteria for Contraceptive Use, 4th edition. *MMWR Morbidity and mortality weekly report*, 59,1-88. (2010)

[5] Berelson, B; Ford Foundation., Population Council. Family planning and population programs; a review of world developments. Chicago: University of Chicago Press; 1966.

[6] Robey, B; Ross, J; Bhushan, I. Meeting unmet need: new strategies. Population reports Series J, *Family planning programs*, 1996, 1-35.

[7] Bogue, DJ. Population perspectives: some views from a sociologist. *Population dynamics quarterly*, 1974, 2, 2.

[8] Bongaarts J. *Population and Development Review*, 17, 293, (1991).

[9] Westoff, CF. *Family planning perspectives*. 10, 173 (1978)

[10] Bradley S. CT; Fishel J., Westoff C. Revising Unmet Need for Family Planning. DHS Analytical Studies ICF International 2012 (Calverton, Maryland, USA) No 25

[11] Jacobstein, R; Curtis, C; Spieler, J; Radloff, S. *Gynaecology and Obstetrics*. 121, Suppl 1, S9,(2013)

[12] United Nations. The Millenium Development Goals Reports. 2013.

[13] Sedgh, G; Singh, S; Hussain, R. Intended and unintended pregnancies worldwide in 2012 and recent trends. *Studies in family planning*. 45, 301(2014).

[14] Westoff, CF. Unmet Need for Modern Contraceptive Methods. DHS Analytical Studies.. ICF International 2012 (Calverton, Maryland, USA.) No. 28

[15] Kessler, K; Goldenberg, SM; Quezada, L. Contraceptive Use, Unmet Need for Contraception, and Unintended Pregnancy in a Context of Mexico-U.S. Migration. Field Actions Science Reports [Online] 2010.

[16] Neukom, J; Chilambwe, J; Mkandawire, J; Mbewe, RK; Hubacher, D. *Contraception*. 83, 447 (2011)

[17] Shelton, J. *Int Fam Plann Perspect*. 27, 152, (2001)

[18] Shelton, JD; Angle, MA; Jacobstein, RA. Medical barriers to access to family planning. *Lancet*. 340,1334 (1992).

[19] Bertrand, J; Hardee, K; Magnani, R; Angle, M. *Int Fam Plann Perspect* 21, 64, (1995).

[20] Finer, LB; Zolna, MR. *American journal of public health.* 104 Suppl 1:S43,(2014).

[21] Finer, LB; Henshaw, SK. *Perspectives on sexual and reproductive health*, 38, 90 (2006).

[22] Sonfield, A; Kost, K; Gold, RB; Finer, LB. *Perspectives on sexual and reproductive health*. 43, 94(2011).

[23] Chandra, A; Martinez, GM; Mosher, WD; Abma, JC; Jones, J. Fertility, family planning, and reproductive health of U.S. women: data from the 2002 National Survey of Family Growth. Vital and health statistics Series 23, Data from the *National Survey of Family Growth.* 1 (2005).

[24] American College of Obstetricans and Gynecologists. ACOG *Obstetrics and gynecology.* 2, 121, 392, (2013).

[25] Chan, LM; Westhoff, CL. Tubal sterilization trends in the United States. *Fertility and sterility.* 94, 1 (2010).

[26] Jones, J; Mosher, W; Daniels, K. *National health statistics reports.* 1(2012)

[27] Secura, GM; Allsworth, JE; Madden, T; Mullersman, JL; Peipert, JF. *American journal of obstetrics and gynecology*. 203,115 e1 (2010).

[28] Secura, GM; Madden, T; McNicholas, C; et al. *The New England journal of medicine. 371, 1316 (2014).*

[29] O'Neil-Callahan, M; Peipert, JF; Zhao, Q; Madden, T; Secura, G. *Obstetrics and gynecology*, 122,1083-91 (2013).

[30] Mestad, R; Secura, G; Allsworth, JE; Madden, T; Zhao, Q; Peipert, JF. *Contraception.* 84, 493 (2011.)

[31] David, PS; Boatwright, EA; Tozer, BS; et al. Hormonal contraception update. *Mayo Clinic proceedings*, 81, 949 (2006).

[32] Lidegaard, O; Lokkegaard, E; Svendsen, AL; Agger, C. *Bmj*, 339, b2890 (2009).

[33] Seeger, JD; Loughlin, J; Eng, PM; Clifford, CR; Cutone, J; Walker, AM. *Obstetrics and gynecology.* 110, 587 (2007).

[34] Amy JJ; Tripathi, V. *Bmj*. 339, b2895 *(*2009).

[35] Lidegaard, O; Nielsen, LH; Skovlund, CW; Skjeldestad, FE; Lokkegaard, E. *Bmj*. 343, d6423 (2011).

[36] Committee on Gynecologic P. ACOG Committee Opinion Number 540 *Obstetrics and gynecology*. 120, 1239 (2012).

[37] Food and Drug Administration. FDA drug safety communication FDA. 2012 (Silver Spring ,MD)

[38] Lidegaard, O; Edstrom, B; Kreiner, S. *Contraception.* 65,187 (2002).

[39] Flegal, KM; Graubard, BI; Williamson, DF; Gail, MH. Excess deaths associated with underweight, overweight, and obesity. *JAMA : the journal of the American Medical Association.* 293,1861 (2005).

[40] Ogden, CL; Carroll, MD; Curtin, LR; McDowell, MA; Tabak, CJ; Flegal, KM. *JAMA : the journal of the American Medical Association.* 295, 1549 (2006).

[41] Canonico, M; Plu-Bureau, G; Lowe, GD; Scarabin, PY. *Bmj.* 336, 1227 (2008).

[42] Pomp, ER; le Cessie, S; Rosendaal, FR; Doggen, CJ. *British journal of haematology.* 139, 289 (2007).

[43] Sidney, S; Petitti, DB; Soff, GA; Cundiff, DL; Tolan, KK; Quesenberry, CP; Jr. *Contraception.* 70, 3 (2004)

[44] National Institutes of Health. Overweight and Obesity Statistics. U.S. Department of Health and Human Services. 2014http:// win.niddk.nih. gov/publications/PDFs/stat904z.pdf

[45] Abdollahi, M; Cushman, M; Rosendaal, FR. *Thrombosis and haemostasis.* 89, 493 (2003).

[46] Stein, PD; Beemath, A; Olson, RE. Obesity as a risk factor in venous thromboembolism. *The American journal of medicine.* 118, 978 (2005).

[47] Speerhas, R. *Cleveland Clinic journal of medicine.* 62, 73 (1995).

[48] Zieman, M; Guillebaud, J; Weisberg, E; Shangold, GA; Fisher, AC; Creasy, GW. *Fertility and sterility.* 77, S13 (2002).

[49] Holt, VL; Cushing-Haugen, KL; Daling, JR. *Obstetrics and gynecology.* 99, 820 (2002).

[50] Edelman, AB; Carlson, NE; Cherala, G; et al. *Contraception*, 80, 119 (2009).

[51] Robinson, JA; Burke, AE. Obesity and hormonal contraceptive efficacy. *Women's health.* 9, 453 (2013).

[52] Trussell, J; Schwarz, EB; Guthrie, K. *Contraception.* 79, 334 (2009).

[53] Tanis, BC; van den Bosch, MA; Kemmeren, JM; et al. *The New England journal of medicine.* 345, 1787 (2001).

[54] Baillargeon, JP; McClish, DK; Essah, PA; Nestler, JE. *The Journal of clinical endocrinology and metabolism*, 90, 3863 (2005).

[55] Lubianca, JN; Moreira, LB; Gus, M; Fuchs, FD. *Journal of human hypertension.* 19, 451 (2005)

[56] American College of Obstetricians and Gynecologists Women's Health Care P. ACOG Practice Bulletin No. 138: *Obstetrics and gynecology.* 122, 706 (2013).

[57] Vandenbroucke, JP; Koster, T; Briet, E; Reitsma, PH; Bertina, RM; Rosendaal, FR. *Lancet.* 344,1453 (1994).

[58] Gompel, A; Piette, JC. *Menopause international*, 13, 65 (2007).

[59] Culwell, KR; Curtis, KM; del Carmen Cravioto, M. *Obstetrics and gynecology*, 114, 341 (2009).

[60] Petri, M; Kim, MY; Kalunian, KC; et al., *The New England journal of medicine* . 353, 2550 (2005).

[61] Sanchez-Guerrero, J; Uribe, AG; Jimenez-Santana, L; et al. *The New England journal of medicine.* 353, 2539 (2005).

[62] Silberstein, SD. *Lancet.* 363, 381 (2004).

[63] Etminan, M; Takkouche, B; Isorna, FC; Samii, A. *Bm.j.* 330, 63(2005).

[64] Schwartz, SM; Petitti, DB; Siscovick, DS; et al. *journal of cerebral circulation.* 29, 2277 (1998).

[65] Edlow, AG; Bartz, D. Hormonal contraceptive options for women with headache: a review of the evidence. *Reviews in obstetrics & gynecology*, 3, 55(2010).

[66] Hauser, WA; Annegers, JF; Kurland, LT. *Epilepsia.* 34, 453 (1993)

[67] Sabers, A; Ohman, I; Christensen, J; Tomson, T. *Neurology.* 61, 570 (2003)

[68] Christensen, J; Petrenaite, V; Atterman, J; et al. *Epilepsia.* 48, 484 (2007).

[69] Manski, R; Dennis, A. *Seizure : the journal of the British Epilepsy Association.* 23, 629 (2014)

[70] Mildvan, D; Yarrish, R; Marshak, A; et al. *Journal of acquired immune deficiency syndromes.* 29, 471 (2002)

[71] El-Ibiary, SY; Cocohoba, JM. *The European journal of contraception & reproductive health care.* (2008), 13, 123-32.

[72] ViiV Healthcare ULC. Telzir (fosamprenavir) Prescribing Information. Montreal, QC February 11, 2014.

[73] Boehringer Ingelheim. Aptivus (tipranavir) Product Monograph. Burlington, ON March 11, 2011.

[74] Hills-Nieminen, C; Foisy, M; Tseng, A. Interactions between Antiretrovirals (ARVs) and Hormonal Contraceptives. 2014. http:// www.hivclinic.ca/main/drugs_interact_files/Oral Contraceptive-int.pdf, accessed November 19, 2014.

[75] Abel, S; Russell, D; Whitlock, LA; Ridgway, CE; Muirhead, GJ. *British journal of clinical pharmacology*, 65, 19 (2008).
[76] Kearney, BP; Mathias, A. *Pharmacotherapy*, 29, 924 (2009).
[77] Robinson, JA; Fox, MC; Jamshidi, R; Trent, M; Anderson, J; Burke, AE. *Obstetrics and gynecology*. 123 Suppl 1:13S (2014)
[78] Killick, SR; Leary, C; Trussell, J; Guthrie, KA; *Human fertility*. 14, 48 (2011)
[79] Mosher, WD; Martinez, GM; Chandra, A; Abma, JC; Willson, SJ. *Advance data*. (2004) 1
[80] Mavranezouli, I. Group LGD, *Human reproduction*. 23, 1338 (2008)
[81] Trussell, J; Leveque, JA; Koenig, JD; et al. *American journal of public health*, (1995), 85, 494
[82] Varney, SJ; Guest, JF. *PharmacoEconomics*. 22, 1141 (2004)
[83] Rak, S; Coffin, J. *The Journal of medical practice management : MPM*. 28, 317 (2013)
[84] Henry, J. Kaiser Family Foundation. Status of state action on the Medicaid expansion decision, of December 11, 2013 at http://kff.org/health-reform/state-indicator/state-activity-around-expanding-medicaid-under-the-affordable-care-act/
[85] Sonfield, A; Pollack, HA. *The Journal of health politics, policy and law*. 38, 373 (2013)
[86] Heberlein, M. Holding Steady, Looking Ahead: Annual Findings of a Fifty-State Survey of Eligibility Rules, Enrollment and Renewal Procedures, and Cost Sharing Practices in Medicaid and CHIP, 2010-2011. Washington, DC: Kaiser Commission on Medicaid and the Uninsured 2011.
[87] Swartz, K. Cost-sharing: effects on spending and outcomes. The Synthesis project Research synthesis report 2010.
[88] Guttmacher Institute, Medicaid family planning expansions, State Policies in Brief 2014, at <http://www.guttmacher.org/ statecenter/ spibs/spib_SMFPE.pdf%3E,
[89] Finer, LB; Sonfield, A; Jones, RK. *Contraception*. 89, 97 (2014)
[90] Hamilton, BE; Ventura, SJ. Birth rates for U.S. teenagers reach historic lows for all age and ethnic groups. *NCHS data brief.* 1 (2012).
[91] Ventura, SJ; Hamilton, BE. *NCHS data brief*, 1 (2011).
[92] Ventura, SJ; Hamilton, BE; Matthews, TJ. *National Vital Statistics System*. 63, 1 (2014).
[93] Santelli, JS; Lindberg, LD; Finer, LB; Singh, S. *American journal of public health*, 97, 150 (2007)

[94] American Academy of Pediatrics Committee on A; Blythe, MJ; Diaz, A. *Pediatrics* . 120,1135 (2007)
[95] Finer, LB; Philbin, JM. *Pediatrics*. 131, 886 (2013)
[96] Martinez, G; Copen, CE; Abma, JC. *National Survey of Family Growth*. 1 (2011)
[97] Centers for Disease C, Prevention. *MMWR Morbidity and mortality weekly report*. 57, 817 (2008)
[98] Eisenberg, D; McNicholas, C; Peipert, JF. *The Journal of adolescent health*. 52, S59 (2013)
[99] Finer, LB; Jerman, J; Kavanaugh, ML. *Fertility and sterility*. 98, 893 (2012)
[100] Committee on Adolescent Health Care Long-Acting Reversible Contraception Working Group TACoO, Gynecologists. Committee opinion no. 539. *Obstetrics and gynecology*. 120, 983 (2012).
[101] Ricketts, S; Klingler, G; Schwalberg, R. *Perspectives on Sexual and Reproductive Health* 46:doi: 10.1363/46e1714. (2014)
[102] Kirby, DB; Laris, BA; Rolleri, LA. *The Journal of adolescent health* . 40, 206 (2007).
[103] Albert, B. With one voice,: America's adults and teens sound off about teen pregnancy. Washington, DC: The National Campaign to Prevent Teen and Unplanned Pregnancy. 2010 http://www. thenationalcampaign.org/resources/pdf/pubs/wov_2010.pdf,
[104] Martino, SC; Elliott, MN; Corona, R; Kanouse, DE; Schuster, MA. *Pediatrics*. 121, e612 (2008).
[105] Gold, R; Sonfeld, A; Richards, CL; Frost, JJ. Next steps for America's family planning program: Leveraging the potential of Medicaid and Title X in an evolving health care system. New York; 2009.
[106] Center for Reproductive Rights. Adolescents' Access to Reproductive Health Services and Information; 2010. http://reproductiverights.org/ en/project/adolescents-access-to-reproductive-health-services-and-information,
[107] Guttmacher Institute, State Policies in Brief As of September 1, 2014. An Overview of Minors' Consent Law. http://www.guttmacher.org/ statecenter/spibs/spib_OMCL.pdf .
[108] Boonstra, HD. 2010a. "Key Questions for Consideration as a New Federal Teen Pregnancy Prevention Initiative Is Implemented." *Guttmacher Policy Review*, 13, no. 1, 2–7. .
[109] LoPresti, AF. *Sex and religion*. Thomson Wadsworth, Toronto (2005)

[110] Schenker, JG. Women's reproductive health: monotheistic religious perspectives. *International journal of gynaecology and obstetrics.* 70, 77 (2000)

[111] Gudorf, CE; Maguire, DC; ed. *Sacred rights: the case for contraception and abortion in world religions* New York: Oxford University Press (2003)

[112] Campbell, F. Birth Control and the Christian Churches. *Population Studies.* Population Investigation Committee, 14, 131 (1960).

[113] LaHaye, T; LaHaye, B. *The act of marriage: the beauty of sexual love.* Grand Rapids, MI: Zondervan(1998)

[114] Ebrahim, AFM. *Abortion, Birth Control and Surrogate Parenting: An Islamic Perspective.* Indianapolis: American Trust Publications; (1998).

[115] Omran, AR; *Family planning in the legacy of Islam.* New York: Routledge(1992).

[116] Poston, L. *Sex and religion.* Toronto,Thomson Wadsworth(2005).

[117] Pennachio, DL. *Med Econ*, 82(9),46 (2005)

[118] Dhami, S; Sheikh, A. *The Western journal of medicine.*173, 352(2000).

[119] Oberneger, CM. *Stud Fam Plann*, (1994), 25, 41-51.

[120] Kridli, SA. *Am J Matern Child Nurs.* 27(3), 178 (2002).

[121] Iyer, S. *J Sci Study Relig*, 41(4), 711 (2002).

[122] Abraham, AS. *The comprehensive guide to medical halachah.* New York:Feldheim Publishers(1996).

[123] Geller, B. *Sex and religion.* Toronto:Thomson Wadsworth (2005).

[124] Feldman, P. *CMAJ.* 35(1), 29 (1992)

[125] Rosner, F. Modern medicine and Jewish ethics. New York: Yeshiva University Press; (1991).

[126] Okun, BS. Religiosity and contraceptive method choice: the Jewish population of Israel. European journal of population *Revue europeenne de demographie*, 16, 109 (2000)

[127] Schenker, JG; Rabenou, V. Family planning: cultural and religious perspectives. *Human reproduction.* 8, 969 (1993).

[128] Srinivas, MN. *Asiaweek.* 53, 59 (1993)

[129] Jain, S. Sacred rights: the case for contraception and abortion in world religions. New York: Oxford University Press(2003).

[130] Planned Parenthood® Federation of America, Inc. Refusal clauses: a threat to reproductive rights.2006 at: http://www.plannedparenthood.org/

[131] Rasmussen, SA, Jamieson DJ. *Clinical Obstetrics and Gynecology.* 55, 487 (2012).

[132] Rasmussen, SA; Jamieson, MD. *New England Journal of Medicine*. 371, 1373 (2014).

[133] World Health Organization. IHR procedures concerning public health emergencies of international concern (PHEIC). http://www.who.int/ihr/procedures/ pheic/en/. accessed August 18, 2014.

[134] World Health Organization. WHO Statement on the Meeting of the International Health Regulations Emergency Committee regarding the 2014 Ebola outbreak in West Africa. http://www.who.int/mediacentre/news/statements/2014/ ebola-20140808/en/. accessed August 20, 2014.

[135] Mupapa, K; Mukundu, W; Bwaka, MA; et al. *The Journal of infectious diseases*, 179, S11 (1999).

[136] American Congress of Obstetricians and Gynecologists. *Obstetrics and gynecology*. 124,1005 (2014).

[137] Caluwaerts, S; Lagrou, D; Van Herp, M; Black, B; Caluwaerts, A; Taybi, A; et al. Guidance paper Ebola Treatment Center: pregnant and lactating women. *Brussels*: *Medecins Sans Frontieres* (2014).

[138] World Health Organization. Ebola Virus Disease. Fact Sheet No. 103. World Health Organization, Geneva (2014).

[139] Mackay, I; Arden, K. *The Lancet Infectious Diseases*. 2014 www.sciencedirect.com/science/article/pii/S1473309001471033. Accessed December 05, 2014.

[140] USAMRIID. Medical management of biological casualties handbook (7th ed.) United States Army Medical Research Institute of Infectious Diseases, Frederick, MD (2011).

[141] Landau, SC; Tapias, MP; McGhee, BT. *Contraception*. 74, 463 (2006)

[142] Landau, S; Besinque, K; Chung, F; et al. *Journal of the American Pharmacists Association*. 49, 43 (2009)

[143] Xu, H; Eisenberg, DL; Madden, T; Secura, GM; Peipert, JF. A*merican journal of obstetrics and gynecology*. 210, e1 (2014)

[144] Rowlands, S. *BJOG : an international journal of obstetrics and gynaecology*. 116, 230 (2009)

[145] Rowlands, S. *The journal of family planning and reproductive health care*. 29, 13 (2003)

[146] Sitruk-Ware, *Human reproduction update*, 12, 169 (2006)

[147] Wildemeersch, D; Janssens, D; Vrijens, M; Weyers, S. *Contraception*. 71, 465 (2005)

[148] Wildemeersch, D; Schacht, E; Wildemeersch, P. *Contraception*. 66, 93 (2002).

[149] Heinemann, K; Saad, F; Wiesemes, M; White, S; Heinemann, L. *Human reproduction*. 20, 549 (2005).

[150] Glasier, AF; Anakwe, R; Everington, D; et al. *Human reproduction*. 15, 646 (2000).

[151] Wang, C; Swerdloff, RS. *American journal of obstetrics and gynecology*. 190, S60 (2004).

[152] American College of Obstetricians and Gynecologists Committee on Long-Acting Reversible Contraception Working. ACOG Committee Opinion no. 450 *Obstetrics and gynecology*. 114, 1434 (2009).

[153] Trussell, J; Wynn, LL. *Contraception*. 77, 1 (2008).

[154] Secura, G. *Minerva ginecologica*. 65, 2712013.

[155] Oakley, D; Bogue, EL. *American journal of public health*. 85, 1526 (1995)

[156] Brindis, C; Davis, L; Clark, MP; Rodine, S. Improving Contraceptive Access for Teens. Advocates for Youth. 1998 at http://www. cachedsimilarwww.themediaproject.com/storage/advfy/documents/com munitiesresponding4.pdf.

In: Contraception
Editor: Alicia Y. Armstrong

ISBN: 978-1-63482-145-2

Chapter 2

Existing Contraceptive Options

Matthew Connell, DO*[*1], *Tiffany Hailstorks, MD*[†2] and *Nneoma Nwachuku, MD*[‡2]

[1]Program in Reproductive and Adult Endocrinology, Eunice Kennedy Shriver National Institute of Child Health and Human Development, National Institutes of Health, Bethesda, MD, US

[2]Howard University Department of Obstetrics and Gynecology Washington, DC, US

Abstract

An estimated 41% of pregnancies are unintended. Globally, 86 million pregnancies were unintended. These unintended pregnancies resulted in 41 million abortions, 33 million unplanned births and 11 million in miscarriages. Nearly half of all pregnancies in the U.S. are unintended, which is defined as any pregnancy either mistimed, unplanned or unwanted .Safe effective contraception is clearly one of the most important areas of reproductive health for women. In this chapter the authors will review the current options for contraception, with special emphasis on efficacy, side effects and patient selection and identify gaps in contraception options.

Correspondence: Alicia Armstrong; ayba55@aol.com
[*] Matthew.t.connell@gmail.com.
[†] thailstorks@gmail.com.
[‡] nnwachuku@gmail.com.

Introduction

Since the dawn of history, women and men have desired the control of when to have a child. Of course, methods used were not always safe or effective. For example, Chinese women would often drink lead and mercury for control of fertility [1]. This would often lead to sterility and death. Other civilizations utilized amulets such as the testicles of a weasel [2], desiccated cat livers, or bones from cats [3]. The earliest writings of contraception come for the Petrie Medical Papyrus from 1950 BC [3]. Within these writings are descriptions for spermicides containing different mixtures of plants with honey or crocodile dung [4]. The Ebers papyrus may have described the first barrier method by describing a paste mixture with a vaginal suppository [3]. Through the years several homemade suppositories and pessaries have been described [5].

Italian anatomist, Gabriello Fallopius, is credited with the first description of a linen sheath to protect the penis in 1564. His goal was not contraception but rather to reduce the transmission of infections. However, it has been regarded as the forerunner to the condom [3]. The story regarding the origin of the word condom has many versions. However most attribute the name from a Dr. Condom; who was an English physician in the 1600s. The most famous story involves Dr. Condom inventing a sheath to prevent pregnancy in response to Charles II annoyance at the number of his illegitimate children. Others believe the work may have originated from the Latin word condon, which means receptacle [6]. The modern era of the condom began in the mid-19th century, where vulcanized rubber made mass production a possibility [7].

During the same time period when condoms became widely used, cervical caps began to appear in the literature. The cervical cap was made of vulcanized rubber and was customized from a wax impression made of the woman's cervix. Soon after, other materials such as impermeable plastic and different metals were used for cervical caps [8]. Later, in 1860 a New York gynecologist, E.B. Foote, published a pamphlet on the use of the cervical cap. This form of contraception gained wide acceptance in Europe [7]. Shortly after the cervical cap, a German gynecologist, C. Haase, wrote the first scientific publication about the diaphragm in 1882. The diaphragm was made of rubber and was sized to fit different vaginal canals [5]. By the mid-1940s, the diaphragm had gained significant popularity with the medical community. This popularity would continue until the 1960s where the oral contraceptive pill and IUD would become more utilized [5, 9].

It has long been thought that the origin of the IUD came from Arab traders placing stones in the uterine cavities of camels to prevent pregnancies during long trips; however these stories are inaccurate [10]. Pessaries, which have been in use since the 1800s, were actually the forerunner of IUDs. These pessaries had a small button structure that would fit over the cervix and were attached to stems that extended up the cervical canal. This pessary was soon found to have some contraceptive benefit. Soon after, in 1902, Hallweg designed a pessary that extended into the uterus. This pessary was sold for self-insertion; however there was a high risk of infection and this pessary quickly earned condemnation from the medical community [7]. The first true IUD was developed in 1909 by Richard Richter. This IUD consisted of a silkworm catgut ring with either a nickel or bronze wire protruding through the cervix [11]. In 1923 Karl Pust combined the button type pessary with Richter's ring and modified the wire by using catgut thread [12]. This was used during The Great War. However, as was the case with similar IUDs, infection remained a frequent problem.

Dr. Ernst Gräfenberg removed the tail as he presumed this was the cause of infection [7]. In 1930 he wrote about the Gräfenberg ring, which was made of coiled silver and gold [13]. During World War II, the Gräfenberg ring fell victim to Nazi party philosophy that was staunchly opposed to contraception [7]. There was little or no use of the IUD during World War II. Following the war, reports from Israel and Japan again sparked interest in the IUD [14, 15]. The use of the IUD flourished in the 1960s and 70s and replaced the cervical cap and diaphragm. However, by the end of the 70s IUD usage markedly declined. This was primarily attributable to the high infection rates seen with the Dalkon Shield. The Dalkon Shield had a multifilament string that allowed ascending bacterial infections [16]. IUD use continued to decline and did not recover until 1995, reflecting the acceptance of the levonorgestrel-releasing intrauterine device [7, 17].

The history of hormonal contraception began in the 1920s. Decades before the approval of the first birth control pill, it had been known that sex hormones were able to suppress ovulation in animal models. In 1921 an Austrian physiologist, Ludwig Haberlandt, found that rabbits and guinea pigs were temporarily sterile after ovaries from pregnant animals were transplanted [18]. He termed this "hormonal sterilization" [19]. Haberlandt is acknowledged as the first to attempt experiments aimed at hormonal contraception [7], and has been referred to as the grandfather of the pill [18]. Haberlandt's work was confirmed by Otfried Otto Fellner; who, in 1922, injected animals with ovarian and placental extracts and reported hormonal sterility [20]. These scientists made the study of progesterone's effect on ovulation possible. In 1937 A.W. Makepeace was able to demonstrate the anti-ovulatory effects of progesterone when injected into rabbits [21]. Up to this point sex steroids had to be isolated from ovaries or gallons of urine. This process was inefficient at best. Russell E. Marker, an organic chemistry professor, changed this process when he was able to manufacture progesterone from a plant root (*Dioscorea mexicana)* [7]. This allowed for mass quantities to be produced cheaply and efficiently.

Gregory Pincus was already well known in the field of experimental biology before starting his work to develop a hormonal contraceptive. In 1934, Pincus successfully reported in vitro fertilization with rabbits. Along with his colleagues Pincus established experimental models that confirmed Makepeace's finding of anti-ovulatory effect of progesterone [22, 23].Much of the early work in hormonal contraception was funded by Margaret Sanger, founder of the Planned Parenthood Federation of America [24]. The more significant grants for research came from Katharine McCormick, who donated up to 2 million dollars [24]. Pincus and Chang's first experiments started in April of 1951. In December of 1953 norethindrone, norethynodrel, and norethandrolone were selected as the three most effective progesterones for inhibiting ovulation. One year later, these three compounds were FDA approved for treatment of menstrual disorders [7].

In collaboration with a physician colleague, John Rock, Dr. Pincus began human trials [7]. John Rock, chief of gynecology and obstetrics at Harvard, had previously met Pincus. They found a mutual interest in reproductive physiology, although Rock was interested in progestational agents [23]. Rock began experiments with 10mg of norethynodrel. By inducing "pseudopregnancy" with the medication, he also noticed ovulation was inhibited [2]. When using a more pure from of norethynodrel, Rock noticed more breakthrough bleeding. It was discovered that the contaminant in the less pure form was mestranol, a synthetic estrogen [18]. This discovery led to the combination of the first birth control pill, Enovid®, which contained 150 micrograms of mestranol and 10 mg of norethynodrel. Clinical trials began in 1956 and in 1960, Enovid® was FDA approved for contraception [18].

Much of the work that has been done since the development of the oral contraceptive pill and the modern IUD have been focused on increasing safety and acceptibility . Newer oral contraceptive formulations have lower doses of estrogen in an effort to decrease the venous thromboembolic risk, and levonorgestrol containing IUDs have been developed which do not have the heavier menstrual bleeding that is associated with earlier intrauterine devices.

Female Non-Hormonal Methods

Scope of the Problem

During the period of 2001-2008, the rate of unintended pregnancy was greater than intended pregnancy for the first time. In 2008 the unintended pregnancy rate was 51% in the United States [25]. Contraceptive non-use and failures of contraception are the two factors that contribute to unintended pregnancies [26]. Nineteen percent of women use contraception inconsistently or incorrectly, and these women account for 43% of all unintended pregnancies. Sixteen percent of women did not practice contraception at all for a month during which they conceived, and these women accounted for 52% of all unintended pregnancies [27].

No Method

Most of the data regarding pregnancy rates in women not using contraception comes from populations who have religious or cultural prohibitions to contraceptive use. Studies of these groups estimate the pregnancy rate to be 85% after one year of unprotected intercourse [28].

Coitus Interruptus

The "withdrawal" method, more formally known as coitus interruptus, is perhaps the oldest form of contraception [29]. This method has several advantages. It may prevent pregnancy when no other methods are available, it is inexpensive if the cost of failures are not included, and it may be combined with other methods to increase efficacy [29]. The prevelance of use is difficult to ascertain. When combined with another method, that other method is counted on most surverys [30]. However, according to the 2002 U.S National Survey of Family Growth, 4% of contracepting women use this method. If withdrawal occurs before ejaculation every time for one year, the failure rate is 4%. However, the more typical use has a failure rate of 22% [28].

There is a paucity of research on this subject. Lack of interest in this method likely stems from several factors, including: preference for modern methods, focusing on methods that prevent pregnancy and sexually transmitted infections, and strongly-held beliefs that pre-ejaculate fluid contains sperm

[30, 31]. There are very few studies that have looked at sperm content in pre-ejaculatory fluid. One previous study found no sperm in pre-ejaculatory fluid [32]. Two small studies looking at HIV virus in pre-ejaculatory fluid found 8 out of 39 men had small clumps of spermatazoa [33, 34]. The largest study to date found 11 out of 27 (41%) subjects produced pre-ejaculatory samples that contained spermatozoa [35]. While impossible to state the pregnancy rate from pre-ejaculatory fluid, based on the current evidence it is not zero.

While withdrawal has several advantages and failure rates approach that of male condom use (perfect use 2% and typical use 18%) [28]; withdrawal does have some limitations. Coitus interruptus requires great self control. Men who prematurely ejaculate should not use this method. Futhermore, individuals wanting protection from STIs should use a different method.

Fertility Awareness-Based Methods

Fertility awareness-based (FAB) methods use a set of physiologic observations that identify fertile days during the menstrual cycle and use this information to avoid intercourse on those days. The fertile period begins 5 days before ovulation and 24 hours after ovulation [36, 37]. These observations rely on five biological pillars: 1. Periodicity of fertility and infertility 2. The occurrence of ovulation once per cycle 3. Lifespan of the ovum, 12-24 hours after ovulation 4. Lifespan of sperm, 3-5 days in the upper genital tract 5. The ability of the individual woman to continually monitor cycle length and related signs and symptoms.

Four different techniques are considered FAB methods and are utilized to predict fertile periods: calendar, basal body temperature, cervical mucus, and symptothermal. The calendar method is the oldest of the group [38, 39]. While the luteal phase is fairly consistent (14 days), the fertile window changes based on the length of the entire menstrual cycle. Before starting the calendar method, a woman should track her cycle lengths for six months and then apply the following rules: subtract 18 days from the shortest experienced cycle to determine the first possible fertile day and subtract 11 days from the longest experienced cycle to determine the last fertile day

Basal body temperature (BBT) is useful for detecting when the fertile period has ended. Temperature is taken daily, preferably in the morning right after waking up. This may be done orally or vaginally. A rise of .5° F that persists for three days indicates that ovulation has taken place [29, 38, 39]. Because the most fertile days of the menstrual cycle are 2 days before ovulation [37], and sperm can live for five days in the upper reproductive tract [29], this method is best used if couples abstain from intercourse from the start of the menstrual cycle until 4 days after the rise in BBT.

Cervical mucus method uses observed changes in the cervical mucus consistency and abundance. These changes are related to changes in estrogen and progesterone levels. The Billings Ovulation Method is the oldest cervical mucus method. Women are tought to monitor mucus daily. Following menses scant mucus should be noted. The next stage notes cervical secretions to be sticky and cloudy appearing. When the cervical mucus becomes stretchy and more abundant, that signifies the start of the fertile window [40]. A simpler method has been devised called the TwoDay Method. This requires a woman to examine herself and ask two questions: "Do I have cervical mucus today?" and "Did I have cervical mucus yesterday?" If the answer to both these questions is no, then the day is deemed safe for unprotected intercourse [41]. This method may be easier as a woman does not have to note changes in mucus and secretions.

Lastly, the symptothermal method combines several of the previously described methods. Along with cervical mucus and BBT, women may also note breast tenderness, back pain, and abdominal pain [29]. Cervical secretions are the foundation of this method and are used to mark the start of the fertile period. BBT is used to mark the end of the fertile period. Other symptoms are used to double-check their findings for defining the fertile window [29, 42].

Efficacy rate from fertility awareness-based methods are difficult to determine. A Cochrane review attempted this, however, significant heterogeneity as well as high drop out rates made it impossible to calculate failure rates [43]. Recently, typical use failure rate has been quoted at 24% for first year use. However, perfect use rates are much better, typically between 3-5%. Symptothermal method has the best perfect use rate at .04% [28]. These rates may vary depending on the population being studied. Age, marital status, and different techniques may affect the pregnancy rate [29]. Overall motivation of the couple changes the pregnancy rate as well [44]. Couples using these methods have a high discontinuation rate at one year (53%) [28]. Many studies looking at various methods have a high drop out rate as well [29]. These methods can often be cumbersome, difficult to teach, and a quarter of patients will become pregnant within one year of its use.

Even though there are high drop out rates, these methods have several advantages. These methods are safe and without side effects. Women can avoid the side effects of hormonal contraception. These methods may be combined with various barrier methods. Discontinuation can lead to pregnancy within a few cycles as couples better understand the fertile period. These benefits must be weighed against several disadvantages. These methods require training that can take several months. The couple must be willing to abstain approximately half the cycle to avoid pregnancy. Intercourse occuring during the fertile window show high pregnancy rates [29]. Some women do not have an increase in BBT with ovulation. Alcohol consumption, late nights, travel, and medication use can lead to inaccurate basal temperature measurement [45]. Women wishing to protect themselves from STIs should choose another method.

Lactational Amenorrhea Method

Lactational amenorrhea method (LAM) uses the physiologic inhibitory effects of prolactin on the hypothalamus to prevent pregnancy. Breast feeding in general is associated with subfertility, however complete anovulation is likely to occur when the following three rules are met:

- Less than six months postpartum
- Breast feeding exclusively
- Amenorrhea

When the following three criteria are met, there is less than a 2% chance of pregnancy [46]. When these specific criteria are not met, pregnancy rates become significantly higher [47].

Diaphragm and Cervical Caps

The diaphragm was the first effective form of contraception in the US that women had control over. However, after the invention of the OCP and IUD, diaphragm use in the US has all but disappeared [7]. Perfect use failure rate is around 6% with typical use failure rate of 12% [28]. Diaphragms are low cost and if properly taken care of will last several years. Diaphragms are completely reversible. Other benefits include reducing the risk of cervical gonorrhea [48], chlamydia, trichomonas [49], and pelvic inflammatory disease [50].

Diaphragms need to be fitted. The largest diaphragm that does not cause discomfort should be used. Patients must be instructed to place the diaphragm before intercourse with spermicide. The diaphragm must be left in for several hours after intercourse. While the diaphragm is cheap, easy to use, and decreases infection risk, there are some side effects. Vaginal mucosa irritation may occur if fitted too tightly. Urinary tract infections are 2 to 3 times more common among users when compared to non users [51].

Cervical caps have similar efficacy to diaphragms. Side effects are similar as well with the exception that cervical caps have less incidence of vaginal mucosa irritation [52]. Cervical caps must be fitted in office. Spermicide must be added as well. Following child birth, a different sized cervical cap may be required. Cervical caps have not been shown to decrease STI transmission like diaphragms.

Spermicides

Spermicides function by forming a physical barrier to prevent sperm movement, and biochemically, by destroying the immobilized sperm [53]. Use of spermicidal agents as a sole method of contraception is increasely rare. Failure rates are quite high (typical use 28% and perfect use 18%, [28]) so most often it is reommended that it be paired with another form of contraception. Spermicides have two components; a chemical agent, the most common being nonoxynol-9, and an excipient. Excipeints come in foams, creams, jellys, films, and suppositories [53].

Spermicides are relatively cheap, easy to use, and do not require a medical visit. This may be beneficial for adolescents and women who have infrequent intercourse. This method is completely reversable and also may be used with breastfeeding. Although initially thought that a reduction in STIs may be possible, several studies have found that spermicides do not protect against gonorrhea, chlamydia, trichomonas, or HIV [54-57]. Furthermore it is thought that spermicides may irritate the vaginal mucosa and increase the risk of STIs [53]. Other disadvantages include allergies, vaginal irritation, and increased risk of urinary tract infection [58, 59].

With the increase in STI and HIV transmission, focus has turned back to spermicides as an antimicrobial and a contraceptive. Currently several forms are being investigated. One such product is tenofovir, an antiretroviral gel. Users of this gel saw a significant reduction in HIV transmission compared to placebo [60]. While this is promising, further work is needed to develop a reliable contraceptive that reduces STI and HIV transmission.

Female Condom

The female condom (FC) is a smooth, loose fitting sheath made of polyurethane. An internal ring at the closed end serves as an internal anchor and covers the cervix. The external ring remains outside of the vagina. In the laboratory, the FC is impermeable to cytomegalovirus and HIV [61]. The FC is fairly durable when being reused [62]. However, the FC has several disadvantages. It can be burdensome, is more expensive than the male condom, and failure rates are slightly higher than the male condom (typical use 21%, perfect use 5% [28]). Despite the disadvantages, this method does allow women the right to control contraception and protects against STIs.

Male Condom

Various condoms are available, however most are made of latex. Condoms function as a physical barrier to prevent pregnancy. The male condom is the only form of contraception proven to prevent the transmission of HIV [63, 64]. Furthermore, latex condoms prevent the transmission of HPV [65]. Condoms are relatively cheap and easy to use. Failure rates are acceptable with typical use 18% and perfect use 2% [28]. There are very few disadvantages of using condoms but include latex allergy, small chance of condoms breaking, need for use every episode of intercourse, and the possibility of improper storage causing deterioration [5].

Best Candidates for Method

While a majority of the methods mentioned can achieve excellent rates of preventing pregnancy, some require much more effort than others. For instance, fertility awareness-based methods can take several months of training and daily monitoring which can make this very burdensome. Furthermore this will limit the availability of sexual activity to only half the cycle. Coitus interruptus requires extreme discipline and can be difficult to continue this method. Furthermore, this method is entirely male dependent. A further drawback to both methods is that neither protect from STIs and should only be used in low risk populations.

Methods that are more supportive of infrequent or unpredictable intercourse would include spermicides and barrier methods. While spermicides are better than no contraception, they should not be used alone as there is a high failure rate. Diaphragm and cervical cap use has all but disappeared in the United States. The male condom achieves the best rates of pregnancy prevention, and as previously discussed, prevents STI transmission. However, if women wish to control their own contraception using barrier methods, they can achieve almost similar rates of pregnancy prevention with the female condom.

Female Hormonal Methods

Combined Oral Contraceptive Pills

Prevention of ovulation is the primary contraceptive mechanism of combined oral contraceptives (COCs) [66]. In this state, there is marked reduction of ovarian estradiol secretion and no progesterone production [67]. Inhibition at the level of the hypothalamus has also been observed by inhibiting the production of GnRH [68]. Some studies have shown lower pituitary responses to exogenous GnRH when taking COCs suggesting that their effect is at the level of the pituitary and the hypothalamus [69, 70]. The progestional agent primarily inhibits LH (preventing ovulation) and the estrogenic compound inhibits FSH (preventing development of a dominant follicle). The first oral contraceptive pills contained 2 to 5 times as much estrogen. Due to unwanted side effects those doses are quite lower today [71]. As a result, more follicular development has been noted in patients taking these lower estrogen containing pills [72,73]. However, progesterone prevents pregnancy by suppressing ovulation. Progesterone also prevents pregnancy by thickening the cervical mucus, impairing tubal motility, and by rendering the endometrium less suitable for pregnancy.

Gonadotropin levels begin to drop immediately after COCs are started. However 7 continuous days are needed to suppress folliculogenesis [74]. Once pill use has been discontinued, gonadotropin levels quickly rise, which accounts for the quick return to fertility upon discontinuation and accidental pregnancy when a pill is missed [75]. The typical regimen for COCs was 21 “active” pills containing estrogen and progesterone followed by 7 “reminder” pills. This was originally done to mimic the normal 28 day menstrual cycle. However, two concerns arose when lower doses of estrogen were used. First, during the off week new follicles begin to develop [76]. There is some concern that the newer low dose pills may allow earlier follicular development during this time period and could lead to more pregnancies [77]. Secondly, while lower doses of estrogen have less metabolic and subjective side effects, more breakthrough bleeding is noted [78]. While almost all of these follicles will not ovulate [79], the knowledge of this increased activity and breakthrough bleeding with lower dose pills lead to the extended regimen of 24 active pills.

A large study with almost 900 patients compared the same COC dose in a 24 day arm versus a 21 day arm. Pregnancy rates were low (.9% for six months of treatment). The 24 day arm had significantly less intracycle bleeding as well as fewer withdrawal bleed days [80]. These findings have been reported in other studies as well [81, 82]. A few studies have looked at ovarian activity suppresion with the extended regimen. These studies all reported that shortening of the hormone free period leads to suppresion of ovarian activity [83-85]. Furthermore, shorter hormone free period leads to greater pituitary-ovarian axis suppresion [86].

While several different extended formulations have been approved, physicians have been using extended continuous regimens for years. Most commonly, this has been done for bleeding disorders, endometriosis, adenomyosis, and menstrual seizures. However, it is becmoing more accepted to take continuous regimens to decrease the number of menstrual cycles in a year. Any formulation of oral contraception may be taken to achieve these effects. Low dose estrogen oral contraceptives have been shown to be very effective in bleeding profiles when taken continuously [87,88,89]. This regimen offers women protection from unwanted pregnancy and offers the benefit of decreased number of bleeding episodes. Furthermore, this regimen has no effect on return to menses or pregnancy once discontinued [90,91].

COCs with perfect use can achieve very low pregnancy rates (.3%) [28]. However, typical use pregnancy rates is around 9% [28]. This difference is mostly due to adherence and consistent use by women rather than an actual failure of the medication [92]. Other issues that involve oral contraceptive failures include medications that interact with oral contraceptives and gastroenteritis [93, 94]. While COC typical use achieves fairly effective pregnancy rates, there are several other advantages to its use. COCs can be obtained for very reasonable cost, can be discontinued at any time, have a quick return to fertility, and have other health benefits as well. While all these benefits make COCs an attractive and popular form of contraceptive, there exist many metabolic side effects.

The majority of metabolic side effects such as lipid profile changes, carbohydrate metabolism, and effects on hormone responsive organs is transient and self limited. The most serious side effects are cardiovascular and are related to estrogen's and progesterone's effect on the coagulation system [95]. The risk of venous thromboembolism (VTE) is dose dependent with the amount of estrogen that is contained within a specific formulation [96]. Several observational studies have determined that low dose estrogen (less than 50 μg) still confers a 3 to 4 fold increased risk of VTE compared to nonpregnant women who are not using oral contraceptives [97-99]. However, the risk of VTE with oral contraception is far less than the risk of VTE with pregnancy [99].

COCs have long been associated with increased risk of arterial thrombosis [100]. This is thought to be related to the thrombotic mechanism and not from atherosclerotic plaque development [101]. While VTE is much more common than arterial occlusions, the consequences are often far more serious; namely myocardial infarction (MI) and thrombotic stroke [101]. Previous case-control studies found an increased risk of cardiovascular disease in oral contraceptive users [102]. However, these women were taking higher doses of sex steroids. Several case-control studies have been performed to exam the relationship between low dose oral contraceptives and the risk of mycardial infarction and stroke [103-107]. These studies concluded that there is no increased risk for MI in healthy patients who are nonsmokers. These studies did find several risk factors including smoking, diabetes, hypertension, abnormal lipid profiles, and family history of stroke or MI.

Thrombotic strokes from oral contraceptives were first reported in 1962 [108]. This was of particular concern for higher dose regimens [109]. Past data is no longer comparable to the newer generations of oral contraceptives. Current evidence suggest that women without risk factor for stroke (i.e., hypertension, smoking, and diabetes) are not at any increased risk [110,111]. There is no increased risk of hemorrhagic stroke and COC use [112]. With all the information reviewed, low dose COC use does not increase the risk of stroke or MI in women who have no predisposing risk factors.

COCs do have metabolic effects on laboratory values but these rarely cause significant issues. These pills can cause mild insulin resistence, however these women have normal glucose tolerance. In general triglycerides and HDL cholesterol increase slightly, while LDL cholesterol descreases [113]. Furthermore the estrogen component increases sex hormone-binding globulin, cortisol-binding globulin, and thyroxine-binding globulin [114, 115]. COCs may raise blood pressure increasing angiotensin levels. Women taking COCs are at slightly higher risk of developing hypertension. The effect appears to be estrogen mediated as progestin only users do not have this risk [116].

Progestin Only Pill

The progestin only pill (POP) contains a small amount of a progestional agent. It must be taken daily in a continuous fashion. Secondary to its low dose, POPs must be taken at the same time every day [117]. The contraceptive effects are mediated more through effects on the endometrium and cervical mucus rather than ovulation suppression [118]. Approximately 60% of patients will ovulate normally while taking POPs [119]. However, one POP containing 75 µg of desogestrel appears to inhibit ovulation more efficiently then other formulations.

POPs are relatively cheap, easy to use, and are easily reversible. Furthermore POPs do not increase the risk of VTE and do not have any metabolic effects on lipids or carbohydrates [120, 121]. While these pills have more beneficial metabolic profiles, there are some disadvantages of POPs. POPs are slightly less effective than COCs. Pregnancies that occur while on POPs are at higher risk of being an ectopic [122]. POPs should be prescribed with caution to latino women who are breast feeding and had gestational diabetes, as POPs were found to increase the risk of type II diabetes 3 fold [123]. Secondary to the unpredictable ovulation, abnormal bleeding can be quite variable and is the main reason why women discontinue this method [124]. Women who experience frequent functional cysts should choose a contraceptive pill with more ovulation suppression as POP users develop significanlty more functional cysts [125]. Lastly, POPs may cause more acne. POPs have been shown to decrease sex hormone-binding globulin allowing more free androgens to circulate [126]. This is the opposite effect of COCs.

Transdermal Contraception

The transdermal contraceptive patch was approved in 2001. It consists of 20 cm^2 matrix that releases continuous small amounts of norelgestromin and ethinyl estradiol [127]. The patch is applied to the skin of the abdomen, buttocks, upper arm, or torso weekly. This is done for three weeks with a patch free week to allow for a withdrawal bleed. The patch is just as effective as oral contraceptive pills [92]. The patch may also be used continuously for 3 months followed by a withdrawal bleed [128]. The most common reactions are intermenstrual bleeding and breast tenderness. This typically resolved after two cycles. Skin reactions occur about 20% of the time [129]. It is unclear if the transdermal contraceptive patch has an increased risk of VTE when compared to oral contraceptive use. Transdermal patch users are exposed to higher levels of estrogen. Several case-control studies have looked at this with mixed results [130, 131, 132]. However, if a difference does exist it is likely very small and still far lower than the risk of VTE during pregnancy.

Transdermal patch has several benefits. Compliance is generally better with the transdermal patch when compared to pill users [129]. This is likely to be due to the convenient dosing. In clinical trials, the need to replace patches for detachment was low (1.8%) [133]. The transdermal patch is completely reversible. The patch should not be used in patients who smoke and are over 35 years old.

Vaginal Contraceptive Ring

The vaginal contraceptive ring releases ethinyl estradiol and etonorgestrel daily. It is a soft flexible ring with an outer diameter of 54 mm and is available in a one-size-fits-all ring. The ring achieves comparable efficacy to the pill [28, 134]. The vaginal ring was associated with higher rates of vaginal discomfort, foreign body sensation, leukorrhea and vaginitis. Despite these side effects, the ring is associated with less irregular bleeding and spotting [134].

Postcoital Contraception

Postcoital contraception, often referred to as emergency contraception, can be hormonal postcoital contraception or involve the use of the Paragard IUD. These methods are used after acts of unprotected intercourse. Originally these methods used high doses of estrogen and were continued for five days. However, there were high rates of nausea and vomiting. This led to the development of an alternative method now called the Yuzpe method.

This method consisted of using an oral contraceptive pill. Two doses of two pills were given 12 hours apart. The Yuzpe method was found to be just as effective and with less side effects [135]. Later on, another hormonal method was developed. This consisted of levonorgestrel .75mg taken twice 12 hours apart. In a large randomized controlled trial levonorgestrel was more efficacious than the Yuzpe method (failure rate of 1.1% versus failure rate of 3.2%, respectively) and had fewer side effects [136]. Regardless of chosen method, either is most effective when taken within 24 hours of the act of intercourse.

The exact mechanism of action has been intensely investigated. Initially it was thought that the endometrium was altered to prevent implanation. However, there is strong evidence now that the mechanism is manifested through delaying or preventing ovulation [137, 138, 139]. Evidence also shows that there is little if any effect on fertilization or implantation [140]. Patients, pharmacists and physicians can be reassured that this treatment is not an abortifacient.

The newest drug for emergency contraception is ulipristal acetate. Ulipristal is a selective progesterone receptor modulator that is very effective for emergency contraception. Ulipristal suppreses follicular growth and can delay ovulation for up to five days. It may be better than progesterone, as ulipristal may even delay ovulation after LH has started to rise [141].

Best Candidates for Method

Hormonal contraceptive methods offer great protection from unwanted pregnancy. The best option for contraception is one that the patient will use reliably and that has the safest side effect profile. This may differ from patient to patient. Taking a thorough history is important as certain conditions, such as hypertension or smoking, may increase the risks of hormonal contraceptive use. A discussion on the risk of VTE should be had with the patient. The risk of VTE is increased when compared to non-contraceptive users, however this risk is still less than the risk of pregnancy.

Recently the CDC created the U.S. Medical Eligibility Criteria for Contraceptive Use. In this document, there are several medical conditions that are covered. Recommendations are made about prescribing contraceptives to patients with certain diagnoses. This can be very helpful for physicians and patients in the decision making process. Furthermore, when deciding on what is best, physicians should counsel patients on the noncontraceptive benefits of oral contraceptives (Figure 3). This will further help patients understand their contraceptive options and will allow them to make an appropriate choice.

It is not surprising that compliance with monthly doses is superior to daily dosing. These methods should be encouraged. Patients with varying work or sleep schedules may benefit from this as they do not have to remember to take the pill at the same time each day. Other patients who say they have difficulty remembering daily medication would also be appropriate candidates. These longer acting preparations like the ring and patch should be prescribed to adolescents as well.

Conflict of interest: None for any authors.

Disclaimer: The views expressed in this manuscript are those of the authors and do not reflect the official policy or position of the National Institutes of Health, Health and Human Services , or the U. S. Government.

References

[1] Skuy, P. (1995). Tales of Contraception: a museum of discovery. *Toronto: Janssen-Ortho Inc.*

[2] Lieberman, J. (1973). A short history of contraception. *American Biology Teacher,* 35(6), 315-318

[3] Speert, H. (2004). Obstetrics and Gynecology: a history and iconography. New York: The Parthenon Publishing Group Belsky, R. (1975, January). *Barrier Methods. Population Reports*, H(3), 37-55.

[4] Belsky, R. (1975, January). *Barrier Methods. Population Reports,* H(3), 37-55.

[5] Batar, I., & Sivin, I. (2010). State-of-the-art of non-hormonal methods of contraception: I. Mechanical barrier contraception. *The European Journal of Contraception and Reproductive Health Care,* 15, 67-88. .

[6] Himes, N. E. (1936). Medical history of contraception. *Baltimore: Williams & Wilkins*

[7] Fritz, M. A., & Speroff, L. (2012). Clincial Gynecologic Endocrinology And Infertility. Philadelphia: *Lippincott Williams & Wilkins.*

[8] Hatcher, R., Trussell, J., Nelson, A., Cates, W., Kowal, D., & Policar, M. (2011). Contraceptive Technology (20 ed.). New York: Ardent Publishing

[9] Tone, A. (2001). Devices and Desires: a history of contraceptives in America. New York: *Hill & Wang*

[10] Thomsen, R. (1988). Camels and the IUD: it was a good story. *Contemporary OB/GYN,* 31(3), pp. 152-61

[11] Richter, R. (1909). Ein mittel zur verhutung der konzeption. D*eutsche* Medizinische Wochenschrift, 85(35), 1525-27.

[12] Pust, K. (1923). Ein brauchbarer frauenshutz. *Deutsche Medizinische Wochenschrift,* 49(29), 952-53.

[13] Gräfenberg, E. (1930). An intrauterine contraceptive method, In: Sanger M, Stone HM, eds. The Practice of Contraception: Proceeding of the 7th International Birth Control Conference, Zurich, Switzerland. Baltimore: *Williams & Wilkins.*

[14] Ishihama, A. (1959). Clincial studies on intauterine rings, especially the present state of contraception in Japan and the experiences in the use of intrauterine rings. *Yokohama Medical Bulletin,* 10(2), 89-105.

[15] Oppenheimer, W. (1959). Prevention of pregnancy by the Graefenberg ring method; a re-evaluation after 28 years' experience. American *Journal of Obstetrics and Gynecology*, 78(2), 446-54.

[16] Tatum, H., Schmidt, F., Phillips, D., McCarty, M., & O'Leary, W. (1975). The Dalkon Shield controversy. Structural and bacteriological studies of IUD tails. *JAMA,* 231(7), 711-7

[17] Mosher, W., & Jones, J. (2010). Use of contraception in the United States: 1982-2008. *Vital and Health Statistics. Series* 23., 29, 1-44.

[18] Dhont, M. (2010). History of oral contraception. The European Journal of Contraception and Reproductive Health Care, 15(S2), S12-18.

[19] Simmer, H. (1970). On the history of hormonal contraception. I. Ludwig Haberlandt (1885-1932) and his concept of "hormonal sterilization". *Contraception,* 1(1), 3-27.

[20] Simmer, H. (1971). On the history of hormonal contraception II. Otfried Otto Fellner (1873-19??) and estrogens as antifertility hormones. *Contraception,* 3(1), 1-20.

[21] Makepeace, A., Weinstein, G., & Friedman, M. (1937). The effect of progestin and progesterone on ovulation in the rabbit. *American Journal of Physiology,* 119, 512-16.

[22] Speroff, L. (2009). A Good Man- Gregory Goodwin Pincus. Portland: *Arnica Publishing, Inc.*

[23] Speroff, L. (Performer). (2011). A Good Man: Gregory Pincus and the Development of Oral Contraception. Portland, Oregon. Retrieved October 16, 2014

[24] Chesler, E. (1992). Woman of Valor: Margaret Sanger and the Birth Control Movement. New York: *Simon and Schuster.*

[25] Finer, L., & Zolna, M. (2014). Shifts in intended and unintended pregnancies in the United States, 2001-2008. *American Journal of Public Health,* 104(Suppl 1), S43-8

[26] Finer, L., & Henshaw, S. (2006). Disparities in rates of unitended pregnancy in the United States, 1994 and 2001. *Perspective on Sexual and Reproductive Health,* 38(2), 90-6

[27] Gold RB, Sonfield A, Richards CL, Frost JJ. Next Steps for America's Family Planning Program: Leveraging the Potential of Medicaid and Title X in an Evolving Health Care System, 2009, Guttmacher Institute: New York.

[28] Trussell, J. (2011). Contraceptive failure in the United States. *Contraception,* 83(5), 397-404.

[29] Freundl, G., Sivin, I., & Batar, I. (2010). State-of-the-art of non-hormonal methods of contraception: IV. Natural family planning. *The European Journal of Contraception and Reproductive Health Care,* 15(2), 113-23

[30] Jones, R., Fennell, J., Higgins, J., & Blanchard, K. (2009). Better than nothing or savvy risk-reduction practice? *The importance of withdrawal. Contraception,* 79(6), 407-10

[31] Rogow, D., & Horowitz, S. (1995). Withdrawal: A review of the literature and an agenda for research. *Studies in Family Planning,* 26(3), 140-53.

[32] Zukerman, Z., Weiss, D., & Orvieto, R. (2003). Does preejaculatory penile secretion originating from Cowper's gland contain sperm? *Journal of Assisted Reproduction and Genetics,* 20(4), 157-9.

[33] Ilaria, G., Jacobs, J., Polsky, B., Koll, B., Baron, P., Maclow, C., Armstrong, D., Schlegel, P. (1992). Detection of HIV-1 DNA sequence in pre-ejaculatory fluid. *Lancet,* 2(8833), 1469.

[34] Pudney, J., Oneta, M., Mayer, K., Seage III, G., & Anderson, D. (1992). Pre-ejaculatory fluid as potential vector for sexual transmission of HIV-1. *Lancet,* 2(8833), 1470.

[35] Killick, S., Leary, C., Trussell, J., & Guthrie, K. (2011). Sperm content of pre-ejaculatory fluid. *Human Fertility,* 14(1), 48-52

[36] Wilcox, A., Weinberg, C., & Baird, D. (1995). Timing of sexual intercourse in relation to ovulation. Effects on the probability of conception, survival of the pregnancy, and sex of the baby. *New England Journal of Medicine,* 333(23), 1517-21.

[37] Wilcox, A., Weinberg, C., & Baird, D. (1998). Post-ovulatory ageing of the human oocyte and embryo failure. *Human Reproduction,* 13(2), 394-7.

[38] Pallone, S., & Bergus, G. (2009). Fertility awareness-based methods: another option for family planning. *Journal of the American Board of Family Medicine,* 22(5), 147-57.

[39] Smoley, B., & Robinson, C. (2012). Natural family planning. *American Family Physician,* 86(10), 924-8.

[40] Billings, J. (1972). Ovulation method of family planning. *Lancet,* 2(7788), 1193-4

[41] Arevalo, M., Jennings, V., Nikula, M., & Sinai, I. (2004). Efficacy of the new TwoDay Method of family planning. *Fertility and Sterility,* 82(4), 885-92.

[42] Frank-Herrmann, P., Heil, J., Gnoth, C., Toledo, E., Baur, S., Pyper, C., . Freundl, G. (2007). The effectiveness of a fertility awarenss based method to avoid pregnancy in relation to a couple's sexual behaviour during the fertile time: a prospective longitudinal study. *Human Reproduction,* 22(5), 1310-19.

[43] Grimes, D., Gallo, M., Grigorieva, V., Nanda, K., & Schulz, K. (2004). Fertility awareness-based methods for contraception. *The Cochrane Database of Systematic Reviews*(4), CD004860.

[44] Fehring, R., Schneider, M., Barron, M. L., & Pruszynski, J. (2013). Influence of motivation on the efficacy of natural family planning. *American Journal of Maternal Child Nursing,* 38(6), 352-8.

[45] Morris, N., Underwood, L., & Easterling, W. J. (1976). Temporal relationship between basal body temperature nadir and leutinizing hormone surge in normal women. *Fertility and Sterility*, 27(7), 780-3

[46] Kennedy, K., Rivera, R., & McNeilly, A. (1989). Consensus statement on the use of breastfeeding as a family planning method. *Contraception,* 39(5), 477-96.

[47] Shaaban, O., & Glasier, A. (2008). Pregnancy during breastfeeding in rural Egypt. *Contraception,* 77(5), 350-4.

[48] Berger, G., Keith, L., & Moss, W. (1975). Prevalence of gonorrhoea among women using various methods of contraception. *British Journal of Venereal Diseases,* 51(5), 307-9.

[49] Rosenberg, M., Davidson, A., Chen, J., Judson, F., & Douglas, J. (1992). Barrier contraceptives and sexually transmitted diseases in women: a comparison of female-dependent methods and condoms. *American Journal of Public Health,* 82(5), 669-74.

[50] Kelaghan, J., Rubin, G., Ory, H., & Layde, P. (1982). Barrier-method contraceptives and pelvic inflammatory disease. *JAMA*, 248(2), 184-7

[51] Fihn, S., Latham, R., Roberts, P., Running, K., & Stamm, W. (1985). Association between diaphragm use and urinary tract infection. *JAMA,* 254(2), 240-5.

[52] Gallo, M., Grimes, D., & Schulz, K. (2002). Cervical cap versus diaphragm for contraception. *The Cochrane Database od Systematic Reviews*(4), CD003551

[53] Batar, I. (2010). State-of-the-art of non-hormonal methods of contraception: II. Chemical barrier contraceptives. *European Journal of Contraception & Reproductive Health Care,* 15(2), 89-95

[54] Richardson, B. A., Lavreys, L., Martin, H. L., Stevens, C. E., Ngugi, Elizabeth N., Mandaliya, K.; Bwayo, J.J., Ndinya-Achola, J.O., Kresiss, J. K. (2001). Evaluation of low-dose nonoxynol-9 gel for the prevention of sexually transmitted diseases: a randomized clinical trial. *Sexually Transmitted Diseases,* 28(7), 394-400.

[55] Roddy, R., Zekeng, L., Ryan, K., Tamoufe, U., & Tweedy, K. (2002). Effect of nonoxynol-9 gel on urogenital gonorrhea and chlamydial infection: a rondomized control trial. *JAMA,* 287(9), 1117-22.

[56] Roddy, R., Zekeng, L., Ryan, K., Tamoufe, U., Weir, S., & Wong, E. (1998). A controlled trial of nonoxynol 9 film to reduce male-to-female transmission of sexually transmitted diseases. *New England Journal of Medicine,* 339(8), 504-10

[57] Van Damme, L., Ramjee, G., Alary, M., Vuylsteke, B., Chandeying, V., Rees, H., Group, C.-1. S. (2002). Effectiveness of COL-1492, a nonoxynol-9 vaginal gel, on HIV-1 transmission in female sex workers a randomised controlled trial. *Lancet,* 360(9338), 971-7

[58] Roddy, R., Cordero, M., Cordero, C., & Fortney, J. (1993). A dosing study of nonoxynol-9 and genital irritation. *International Journal of STD & AIDS,* 4(3), 165-70

[59] Hooton, T., Scholes, D., Hughes, J., Winter, C., Roberts, P., Stapleton, A., Stamm, W. (1996). A prospective study of risk factors for symptomatic urinary tract infection in young women. *New England Journal of Medicine,* 335(7), 468-74.

[60] Abdool Karim, Q., Abdool Karim, S., Frohlich, J., Grobler, A., Baxter, C., Mansoor, L., Kharsany, A. B. M., Sibeko, S., Mlisana, K. P., Omar, Z., Gengiah, T. N., Maarschalk, S., Arulappan, N., Mlotshwa, M., Morris, L., Taylor, D., on behalf of the CAPRISA 004 Trial Group (2010). Effectiveness and safety of tenofovir gel, an antiretroviral microbicide, for the prevention of HIV infection in women. *Science,* 329(5996), 1168-74

[61] Drew, W., Blair, M., Miner, R., & Conant, M. (1990). Evaluation of the virus permeability of a new condom for women. *Sexually Transmitted Diseases,* 17(2), 110-2.

[62] Beksinska, M., Rees, H., Dickson-Tetteh, K., Mgogi, N., Kleinschmidt, I., & McIntyre, J. (2001). Structural integrity of the female condom after

multiple uses, washing, drying, and re-lubrication. *Contraception,* 63(1), 33-6.

[63] de Vencenzi, I., & HIV, E. S. (1994). A longitudinal study of human immunodeficiency virus transmission by heterosexual partners. *New England Journal of Medicine,* 331(6), 341-6.

[64] Davis, K., & Weller, S. (1999). The effectiveness of condoms in reducing heterosexual transmission of HIV. *Family Planning Perspectives,* 31(6), 272-9.

[65] Winer, R., Hughes, J., Feng, Q., O'Reilly, S., Kiviat, N., Holmes, K., & Koutsky, L. (2006). Condom use and the risk of genital human papillomavirus infection in young women. *New England Journal of Medicine,* 354(25), 2645-54.

[66] Rivera, R., Yacobson, I., & Grimes, D. (1999). The mechanism of action of hormonal contraceptives and intrauterine contraceptive devices. *American Journal of Obstetrics and Gynecology,* 181(5), 1263-9.

[67] Mishell, D. J., Kletzky, O., Brenner, P., Roy, S., & Nicoloff, J. (1977). The effect of contraceptive steriods on hypothalamic-pituitary function. *American Journal of Obstetrics and Gynecology,* 128(1), 60-74.

[68] Kastin, A., Schally, A., Gual, C., & Arimura, A. (1972). Release of LH and FSH after administration of synthetic LH-releasing hormone. *Journal of Clinical Endocrinology and Metabolism*, 34(4), 753-6.

[69] Scott, J., Brenner, P., Kletzky, O., & Mishell, D. J. (1978). Factors affecting pituitary gonadotropin function in users of oral contraceptive steroids. *American Journal of Obstetrics and Gynecology*, 130(7), 817-21.

[70] Robyn, C., Schondorf, H., Jurgensen, O., Dericks-Tan, J., & Taubert, H. (1974). Oral contraception can decrease the pituitary capacity to release gonadotrphins in response to synthetic LH-releasing-hormone. *Archiv Fur Gynakologie,* 216(1), 73-80.

[71] Petitti, D. (2003). Clincial practice. Combination estrogen-progestin oral contraceptives. *New England Journal of Medicine,* 349(15), 1443-50

[72] Baerwald, A., Olatunbosun, O., & Pierson, R. (2004). Ovarian follicular development is initiated during the hormone-free interval of oral contraceptive use. *Contraception*, 70(5), 371-7.

[73] Crosignani, P., Testa, G., Vegetti, W., & Parazzini, F. (1996). Ovarian activity during regular oral contraceptive use. *Contraception,* 54(5), 271-3.

[74] Molloy, B., Coulson, K., Lee, J., & Watters, J. (1985). “Missed pill” conception: fact or fiction? *British Medical Journal*, 290(6480), 1474-5.

[75] Elstein, M., Morris, S., Groom, G., Jenner, D., Scarisbrick, J., & Cameron, E. (1976). Studies on low-dose oral contraceptives: cervical mucus and plasma hormone changes in relation to circulating D-norgestrel and 17 alpha ethynyl-estradiol concentrations. *Fertility and Sterility,* 27(8), 892-9.

[76] Killick, S., Eyong, E., & Elstein, M. (1987). Ovarian follicular development in oral contraceptive cycles. *Fertility and Sterility,* 48(3), 409-13.

[77] Wiebe, E., & Trussell, J. (2009). Contraceptive failure related to estimated cycle day of conception relative to the start of the last bleeding episode. *Contraception*, 79(3), 178-81.

[78] Law, B. (1979). Advantages and disadvantages of low-dose oral contraceptives. *International Journal of Gynaecology and Obstetrics,* 16(6), 556-60

[79] van Heusden, A., & Fauser, B. (1999). Activity of the pituitary-ovarian axis in the pill-free interval during use of low-dose combined oral contraceptives. *Contraception,* 59(4), 237-43.

[80] Nakajima, S., Archer, D., & Ellman, H. (2007). Efficacy and safety of a new 24-day oral contraceptive regimen of norethindrone acetate 1mg/ethinyl estradiol 20 micro g (Loestrin 24 Fe*). Contraception,* 75(1), 16-22.

[81] Endrikat, J., Cronin, M., Gerlinger, C., Ruebig, A., Schmidt, W., & Dusterber, B. (2001). Open, multicenter comparison of efficacy, cycle control, and tolerability of a 23-day oral contraceptive regimen with 20 microg ethinyl estradiol and 75 microg gestodene and a 21-day regimen with 20 microg ethinyl estradiol and 150 microg desogesterl. *Contraception,* 64(3), 201-7.

[82] Endrikat, J., Cronin, M., Gerlinger, C., Ruebig, A., Schmidt, W., & Dusterberg, B. (2001). Double-blind, multicenter comparison of efficacy, cycle control, and tolerability of a 23-day versus 21-day low-dose oral contraceptive regimen containing 20 microg ethinyl estradiol and 75 microg gestodene. *Contraception,* 64(2), 99-105.

[83] Spona, J., Elstein, M., Feichtinger, W., Sullivan, H., Ludicke, F., Muller, U., & Desterberg, B. (1996). Shorter pill-free interval in combined oral contraceptives decreases follicular development. *Contraception,* 54(2), 71-7.

[84] Sullivan, H., Furniss, H., Spona, J., & Elstein, M. (1999). Effect of 21-day and 24-day oral contraceptive regimens containing gestodene (60

microg) and ethinyl estradiol (15 microg) on ovarian activity. *Fertility and Sterility,* 72(1), 115-20.

[85] Klipping, C., Duijkers, I., Trummer, D., & Marr, J. (2008). Suppression of ovarian activity with a drospirenone-containing oral contraceptive in a 24/4 regimen. *Contraception,* 78(1), 16-25.

[86] Willis, S., Kuehl, T., Spiekerman, A., & Sulak, P. (2006). Greater inhibition of the pituitary-ovarian axis in oral contraceptive regimens with a shortened hormone-free interval. *Contraception,* 74(2), 100-3.

[87] Kwiecien, M., Edelman, A., Nichols, M., & Jensen, J. (2003). Bleeding patterns and patient acceptability of standard or continuous dosing regimens of a low-dose oral contraceptive: a randomized trial. *Contraception,* 67(1), 9-13.

[88] Edelman, A., Koontz, S., Nichols, M., & Jensen, J. (2006). Continuous oral contraceptives: are bleeding patterns dependent on the hormone given? *Obstetrics and Gynecology,* 107(3), 657-65.

[89] Teichmann, A., Apter, D., Emerich, J., Greven, K., Klasa-Mazurkiewicz, D., Melis, G., Spielmann, D. (2009). Continuous, daily levonorgestrel/ ethinyl estradiol vs. 21-day, cyclic levonorgestrel/ethinyl estradiol: efficacy, safety and bleeding in a randomized, open-label trial. *Contraception,* 80(6), 504-11

[90] Archer, D., Kovalevsky, G., Ballagh, S., & Grubb, G. (2009). Ovarian activity and safety of a novel levonorgestrel/ethinyl estradiol continuous oral contraceptive regimen. *Contraception*, 80(3), 245-53.

[91] Davis, A., Kroll, R., Soltes, B., Zhang, N., Grubb, G., & Constantine, G. (2008). Occurrence of menses or pregnancy after cessation of a continuous oral contraceptive. *Fertility and Sterility,* 89(5), 1059-63.

[92] Trussell, J. (2009). Understanding contraceptive failure. *Best Practice & Research Clinical Obstetrics and Gynecology,* 23(2), 199-209.

[93] Sparrow, M. (1987). Pill method failure. *New Zealand Medical Journal,* 100(818), 102-5.

[94] Hansen, T., & Lundvall, F. (1997). Factors influencing the reliability of oral contraceptives. *Acta Obstetricia Et Gynecologica Scandinavica,* 76(1), 61-4.

[95] Oral Contraceptive and Hemostasis Study Group. (2003). The effects of seven monophasic oral contraceptive regimens on hemostatic variables: conclusion from a large randomized multicenter study. *Contraception,* 67(3), 173-85.

[96] Gerstman, B., Piper, J., Tomita, D., Ferguson, W., Stadel, B., & Lundin, F. (1991). Oral contraceptive estrogne dose and the risk of deep venous

thromboembolic disease. *American Journal of Epidemiology,* 133(1), 32-7

[97] Contraception, W. H. (1995). Effect of different progestagens in low oestrogen oral contraceptives on venous thromboesmbolic disease. *Lancet,* 346(8990), 1582-88.

[98] World Health Oganization Collaborative Study of Cardiovascular Disease and Steroid Hormone Contraception. (1995). Venous thromboembolic disease and combined oral contraceptives: results of international multicentre case-control study. *Lancet,* 346(8990), 1575-1582.

[99] Lidegaard, O., Edstrom, B., & Kreiner, S. (2002). Oral contraceptives and venous thromboembolism: a five-year national case-control study. *Contraception,* 65(3), 187-96.

[100] Lalude, O. (2013). Risk of cardiovascular events with hormonal contraception: insights from the Danish cohort study. *Current Cardiology Reports,* 15(7), 374-82.

[101] Lidegaard, O., Lokkegaard, E., Jensen, A., Skovlund, C., & Keiding, N. (2012). Thrombotic stroke and myocardial infarction with hormonal contraception. *New England Journal of Medicine,* 366(24), 2257-66.

[102] Stampfer, M., Willett, W., Colditz, G., Speizer, F., & Hennekens, C. (1988). A prospective study of past use of oral contraceptive agents and risk of cardiovascular diseases. *New England Journal of Medicine,* 319(20), 1313-7.

[103] Sidney, S., Petitti, D., Quesenberry, C. J., Klatsky, A., HK, Z., & Wolf, S. (1996). Myocardial infarction in users of low-dose oral contraceptives. *Obstetrics and Gynecology,* 88(6), 939-44.

[104] Lewis, M., Heinemann, L., Spitzer, W., MacRae, K., & Bruppacher, R. (1997). The use of oral contraceptives and the occurrence of acute myocardial infarction in young women. Results from the Transnational Study on Oral Contraceptives and the Health of Young Women. *Contraception,* 56(3), 129-40.

[105] Lewis, M., Spitzer, W., Heinemann, L., MacRae, K., & Bruppacher, R. (1997). Lowered risk of dying of heart attack with third generation pill may offset risk of dying of thromboembolism. *British Medical Journal,* 315(7109), 679-80.

[106] Dunn, N., Thorogood, M., Faragher, B., de Caestecker, L., MacDonald, T., McCollum, C., Thomas, S. & Mann, R. (1999). Oral contraceptives and myocardial infarction: results of the MICA case-control study. *British Medical Journal*, 318(7198), 1579-83.

[107] Rosenberg, L., Palmer, J., Rao, R., & Shapiro, S. (2001). Low-dose oral contraceptive use and the risk of myocardial infarction. *Archives of Internal Medicine,* 161(8), 1065-70

[108] Lorentz, I. (1962). Parietal lesion and "Enavid". *British Medical Journal,* 2(5313), 1191.

[109] Collaborative Group for the Study of Stroke in Young Women. (1975). Oral contraceptives and stroke in young women: associated risk factors. *JAMA*, 231(7), 718-22.

[110] Siritho, S., Thrift, A., McNeil, J., You, R., Davis, S., Donnan, G., & Group, M. R. (2003). Risk of ischemic stroke among users of the oral contraceptive pill: the Melbourne risk factor study (MERFS) group. *Stroke,* 34(7), 1575-80

[111] Wee-Shian, C., Ray, J., Wai, E., Ginsburg, S., Hannah, M., Corey, P., & Ginsberg, J. (2004). Risk of stroke in women exposed to low-dose oral contraceptives. *Archives of Internal Medicine,* 164(7), 741-747.

[112] Peragallo Urrutia, R., Coeytaux, R., McBroom, A., Gierisch, J., Havrilesky, L., Moorman, P Myers, E. (2013). Risk of acute thromboembolic events with oral contraceptive use: a systematic review and meta-analysis. *Obstetrics and Gynecology,* 122(2 Pt 1), 380-9.

[113] Krauss, R., & Burkman, R. (1992). The metabolic impact of oral contraceptives. *American Journal of Obstetrics and Gynecology,* 167(4 Pt 2), 1177-84.

[114] Wiegratz, I., Kutschera, E., Lee, J., Moore, C., Mellinger, U., Winkler, U., & Kuhl, H. (2003). Effect of four oral contraceptives on thyroid hormones, adrenal and blood pressure parameters. *Contraception,* 67(5), 361-6.

[115] Cullberg, G., Hamberger, L., Mattsson, L., Mobacken, H., & Samsioe, G. (1985). Effects of a low-dose desogestrel-ethinylestradiol combination on hirsutism, androgens and sex hormone binding globulin in women with a polycystic ovary syndrome. *Acta Obstetricia et Gynecologica Scandinavica,* 64(3), 195-202.

[116] Wilson, E., Cruickshank, J., McMaster, M., & Weir, R. (1984). A prospective controlled study of the effect on blood pressure of contraceptive preparations containing different types and dosages of progestogen. *British Journal of Obstetrics and Gynaecology*, 91(12), 1254-60.

[117] Brooms, M., & Fotherby, K. (1990). Clinical experience with the progestogen-only pill. *Contraception,* 42(5), 489-95.

[118] Chi, I. (1993). The safety and efficacy issues of progestin-only oral contraceptives-An epidemiologic perspective. *Contraception,* 47(1), 1-21.

[119] Rice, C., Killick, S., Dieben, T., & Coelingh Bennink, H. (1999). A comparison of the inhibition of ovulation achieved by desogestrel 75 μg and levonorgestrel 30 μg daily. *Human Reproduction*, 14(4), 982-985.

[120] Godsland, I., Crook, D., Simpson, R., Proudler, T., Felton, C., Lees, B., Anyaoku, V., Devenport, M. & Wynn, V. (1990). The effects of different formulations of oral contraceptive agents on lipid and carbohydrate metabolism. *New England Journal of Medicine,* 323(20), 1375-81.

[121] Hall, K., Trussell, J., & Schwarz, E. (2012). Progestin-only contraceptive pill use among women in the United States. *Contraception,* 86(6), 653-8.

[122] Furlong, L. (2002). Ectopic pregnancy risk when contraception fails. A review. *Journal of Reproductive Medicine*, 47(11), 881-5.

[123] Kjos, S., Peters, R., Xiang, A., Thomas, D., Schaefer, U., & Buchanan, T. (1998). Contraception and the risk of type 2 diabetes mellitus in Latina women with prior gestational diabetes mellitus. *JAMA,* 280(6), 533-8.

[124] Kovacs, G. (1996). Progestogen-only pills and bleeding disturbances. *Human Reproduction,* 11(Suppl 2), 20-3.

[125] Tayob, Y., Adams, J., Jacobs, H., & Guillebaud, J. (1985). Ultrasound demonstration of increased frequency of functional ovarian cysts in women using progestogen-only oral contraception. *British Journal of Obstetrics and Gynaecology,* 92(10), 1003-9.

[126] Song, S., Chen, J., Lu, C., Yang, P., Yang, Q., Fan, B., . . . Fotherby, K. (1993). Effects of different doses of norethisterone on ovarian function, serum sex hormone binding globulin and high density lipoprotein-cholesterol. *Contraception,* 47(6), 527-37.

[127] Abrams, L., Skee, D., Natarajan, J., Wong, F., & Lasseter, K. (2001). Multiple-dose pharmacokinetics of a contraceptive patch in healthy women participants. *Contraception,* 64(5), 267-94.

[128] Stewart, F., Kaunitz, A., Laguardia, K., Karvois, D., Fisher, A., & Friedman, A. (2005). Extended use of transdermal norelgestromine/ ethinyl estradiol: a randomized trial. *Obstetrics and Gynecology,* 105(6), 1389-96.

[129] Audet, M., Moreau, M., Koltun, W., Waldbaum, A., Shangold, G., Fisher, A., Group, O. E. (2001). Evaluation of contraceptive efficacy and

cycle control of a transdermal contraceptive patch vs an oral contraceptive: a randomized controlled trial. *JAMA,* 285(18), 2347-54

[130] Jick, S., Kaye, J., Russmann, S., & Jick, H. (2006). Risk of nonfatal venous thromboembolism in women using a contraceptive transdermal patch and oral contraceptives containing norgestimate and 35 microg of ethinyl estradiol. *Contraception,* 73(3), 223-8.

[131] Jick, S., Kaye, J., Li, L., & Jick, H. (2007). Further results on the risk of nonfatal venous thromboembolism in users of the contraceptive transdermal patch compared to users of oral contraceptives containing norgestimate and 35 microg of ethinyl estradiol. *Contraception,* 76(1), 4-7.

[132] Jick, S., Hagberg, K., Hernandez, R., & Kaye, J. (2010). Postmarketing study of ORTHO EVRA and levonorgestrel oral contraceptives containing hormonal contraceptives with 30 mcg of ethinyl estradiol in relation to nonfatal venous thromboembolism. *Contraception,* 81(1), 16-21

[133] Zacur, H., Hedon, B., Mansour, D., Shangold, G., Fisher, A., & Creasy, G. (2002). Integrated summary of Ortho Evra/Evra contraceptive patch adhesion in varied climates and conditions. *Fertility and Sterility*, 77(2 Suppl 2), S32-5.

[134] Roumen, F. (2007). The contraceptive vaginal ring compared with the combined oral contraceptive pill: a comprehensive review of randomized controlled trials. *Contraception,* 75(6), 420-9.

[135] Yuzpe, A., Smith, R., & Rademaker, A. (1982). A multicenter clinical investigation employing ethinyl estradiol combined with dl-norgestrel as postcoital contraceptive agent. *Fertility and Sterility,* 37(4), 508-13.

[136] Task Force on Postovulatory Methods of Fertility Regulation. (1998). Randomised controlled trial of levonorgestrel versus the Yuzpe regimen of combined oral contraceptives for emergency contraception. *The Lancet,* 352(9126), 428-433.

[137] Croxatto, H., Fuentealba, B., Brache, V., Salvatierra, A., Alvarez, F., Massai, R., . . . Faundes, A. (2002). Effects of the Yuzpe regimen, given during the follicular phase, on ovarian function. *Contraception,* 65(2), 121-8.

[138] Marions, L., Hultenby, K., Lindell, I., Sun, X., Stabi, B., & Gemzell Danielsson, K. (2002). Emergency contraception with mifepristone and levonorgestrel: mechanism of action. *Obstetrics and Gynecology,* 100(1), 65-71.

[139] Lalitkumar, P., Lalitkumar, S., Meng, C., Stavreus-Evers, A., Hambiliki, F., Bentin-Ley, U., & Gemzell-Danielsson, K. (2007). Mifepristone, but not levonorgestrel, inhibits human blastocyst attachment to an in vitro endometrial three-dimensional cell culture model. *Human Reproduction,* 22(11), 3031-3037.
[140] Novikova, N., Weisberg, E., Stanczyk, F., Croxatto, H., & Fraser, I. (2007). Effectiveness of levonorgestrel emergency contraception given before or after ovulation--a pilot study. *Contraception,* 75(2), 112-8.
[141] Glasier, A., Cameron, S., Fine, P., Logan, S., Casale, W., Van Horn, J., Gainer, E. (2010). Ulipristal acetate versus levonorgestrel for emergency contraception: a randomized non-inferiority trial and meta-analysis. *Lancet,* 375(9714), 555-62.

Male Contraception

While options for reversible contraception for women have rapidly expanded over the past century, the development of new male contraceptive options has been very limited. The arrival of pills, patches, rings and LARC methods for women have made highly effective and safe options for contraception widely available, however, the paucity of male-initiated contraceptive methods require the female partner to be responsible for the couple's contraceptive method. There is evidence to suggest that men would in fact welcome the opportunity to be more involved in making family planning decisions. A 2002 multinational survey supports the idea that men do take part in contraceptive decision-making, and they desire a greater role [1]. The existing male-directed methods (i.e., coitus interruptus, condoms, and vasectomy), account for less than one third of contraceptive methods used by couples in the United States [2]. Expanding male contraceptive options would most likely increase this number. The World Health Organization has, in fact, recently identified the need for effective male contraception as a priority within the greater global discussion of family planning [3].

In the following section, current options and their limitations will be reviewed. Current reversible methods of male contraception have high typical use failure rates. Vasectomy, while effective, remains an unattractive option for men desiring future fertility. The challenge is identifying a reversible male contraceptive method that is comparable to other female methods in regards to efficacy, tolerable side effect profile, and ease of use.

The most commonly used male contraceptive, the condom, is a barrier method which prevents fertilization through the prevention of sperm transport through the female reproductive tract. The estimated prevalence of use in the developed world is 18%. [4] The advantages of the male condom include availability without the need for a prescription, a lack of serious side effects, affordability, and STI prevention. [5] There are a number of significant disadvantages, however, which include the requirement for the male partner to have responsibility for the correct application and consistent use. Even with precision and consistency in application there is an average failure rate of 18% [6].

Vasectomy, also a form of male sterilization, blocks the physical transport of sperm via the surgical interruption of the vas deferens. Although it is considered an irreversible form of male contraception, it does not immediately produce sterility. An advantage of the vasectomy compared to similar surgical procedures in women, include its lower cost, safety, no need for general anesthesia, and a more rapid recovery. The early failure rates are low with one review of the literature demonstrating an early failure rate (spermatozoa persisting up to four months) in < 1% [7]. The effectiveness and complication rate are highly variable and dependent on the experience of the surgeon. The most common adverse complications include hematomas, infection, sperm granulomas, epididymitis, orchitis, and congestive epididymitis, which occurred in 1-6% of subjects [7]. The risk of pregnancy post-vasectomy is estimated to be 1 in 2,000 men. Men who choose vasectomy as permanent contraception require a post-vasectomy semen analysis (PVSA) to confirm sterility, which is recommended between eight to sixteen weeks post procedure [8]. In a review by Griffin et al. they reported azoospermia in only 80% of subjects and at median time of three months and 20 ejaculations [9]. A vasectomy is considered a failure if motile sperm are visualized on PVSA six months post-procedure. Even in those demonstrating azoospermia or rare non-motile sperm on PVSA, a repeat vasectomy may be necessary in up to 1% of subjects [7].

Despite some limitations, worldwide, vasectomy is one of the most commonly chosen contraceptive methods. A national survey of family growth conducted by the CDC from 2006-2010 found that male sterilization ranked fourth among the most common methods of contraception in the United States at 10%. [7]

Current reversible methods of male contraception have high typical use failure rates as outlined above. Vasectomy, while effective, remains an unattractive option for men desiring future fertility. The quest remains for a reversible male contraceptive method that is comparable to other female methods in regards to efficacy, tolerable side effect profile, and ease of use. Several hormonal preparations designed to achieve reversible azoospermia/oligospermia are currently in clinical trials. Additionally, non-hormonal regimens have been identified as potential candidates for male contraception. Lastly, efforts are being made to enhance the reversibility of surgical approaches, without compromising its intended goal. In the following chapter new technologies, including hormonal methods of male contraception will be reviewed.

References

[1] Heinemann K, Saad F, Wiesemes M, White S, Heinemann L. Attitudes toward male fertility control: results of a multinational survey on four continents. *Human Reproduction*. 2005 Feb;20(2):549-56

[2] Piccinino LJ, Mosher WD. Trends in contraceptive use in the United States: 1982-1995. *Family Planning Perspective*. 1998 Jan-Feb;30(1):4-10, 46

[3] WHO/PAHO (2002) Programming for Male Involvement in Reproductive Health. *Report of the WHO regional advisors in reproductive health.* WHO, Washington DC, USA, pp. 1–179

[4] World Contraceptive Patterns. (2013). United Nations Department of Economic and Social Affairs, Population Division. http://www.un.org/en/development/desa/population/publications/pdf/family/worldContraceptivePatternsWallChart2013.pdf (Accessed October 1, 2014).

[5] Batar, I and I. Sivin (2010). State-of-the-art of non-hormonal methods of contraception: I. mechanical barrier contraception. The European Journal of Contraception and Reproductive Health Care. 15:67-88

[6] Reproductive Health – Contraception (2013). Centers for Disease Control and Prevention. http://www.cdc.gov/reproductivehealth/unintendedpregnancy/contraception.htm. (Accessed October 2, 2014).

[7] Schwingl and Guess. (2000). Safety and effectiveness of vasectomy. *Fertility and Sterility*. 73(5): 923-936

[8] Sharlip ID, Belker, AM, Honig S, Labrecque M, Marmar JL, Ross LS, Sandlow JI, and DC Soka. (2012) Vasectomy. American Urological Association. http://www.auanet.org/education/guidelines/vasectomy.cfm (Accessed October 4, 2014).

[9] National Survey of Family Growth. Centers for Disease Control and Prevention. (2012). http://www.cdc.gov/nchs/data/factsheets/factsheet_nsfg.htm (Accessed October 4, 2014).

LARC

Background

Unintended pregnancy typically arises from the nonuse of contraception, or the failure of a contraceptive method. It is estimated that 7.4% of sexually active women of reproductive age do not use any form of contraception. Of reproductive aged women, 23% use permanent sterilization while the remainder use a reversible form of contraception providing temporary prevention of fertility. Contraception embodies a preventive health measure that when used appropriately, can aid in effectively preventing unintended or unwanted pregnancy. When deciding on the proper contraceptive method, it is necessary to evaluate the advantages and disadvantages of each method in order to determine which method is most appropriate for the patient [1, 2]. This section will review long acting reversible contraceptives.

Contraceptive methods which do not require daily patient compliance often have user failure rates that are close to ideal use rates. These methods are often categorized as "highly effective" methods. Long acting reversible contraception (LARC), including the intrauterine device (system) and the implant, are the most effective reversible contraceptive options. LARC methods are safe and highly effective at preventing pregnancy, with failure rates comparable to sterilization. Their efficacy is attributed to the limited requirements necessary by the patient once the device is inserted, as well minimal use behaviors required for maintenance. LARC uptake in the United States for women aged 15-44 remains low despite widespread use internationally. As of 2009, only 8.5% of women reported using the IUD or implant [3].

Intrauterine Systems

There are three different types of intrauterine systems available for use in the United States. The copper IUD (Copper T380A) is a non-hormonal T-shaped device. The device is comprised of polyethylene wrapped with copper wire around the stem and arms. The copper IUD is FDA approved for 10 years, with a one-year failure rate of 0.8 per 100 women [4].

The two hormonal options include the Mirena and Skyla intrauterine systems. These two devices are also T-shaped, and contain a polydimethylsiloxane sleeve that contains levonorgestrel on the stem. The Mirena T-shaped body design is 32mm x 32 mm, and contains 52 mg of levonorgestrel that is dispersed at a rate of 20micrograms/day. The rate progressively declines over the lifetime of the device with it reaching half of the initial rate after 5 years. Mirena is FDA approved for 5 years, but can last for 7 years, and perhaps up to 10 years [5, 6]. The one-year failure rate for the Mirena is 0.2 per 100 women [7]. This device is approved for contraception and the management of menorrhagia.

The Skyla intrauterine system was FDA approved in 2013 for the prevention of pregnancy for up to 3 years. The flexible T-shaped body is 28mm x 30mm. The insertion device is 3.8mm in diameter compared to the Mirena insertion device, which is 4.4mm. Skyla allows for a smaller insertion device and system, offering an appealing option for nulliparous women. A smaller device permits an easier insertion and potentially less discomfort during the insertion process. The Skyla intrauterine system contains 13.5mg of levonorgestrel released at approximately 14mcg/day, with the rate decreasing progressively to 5mcg/day after 3 years. The failure rate for Skyla is 0.4% at one year and 0.9% cumulative over 3 years [8, 9].

The contraceptive action of the intrauterine systems is localized to the uterine cavity. Ovulation is not affected, and the IUD will not induce an abortion. The presence of IUDs creates an intrauterine environment that is spermicidal [10]. The copper IUD creates a sterile inflammatory response thus prohibiting fertilization of the ovum by the sperm. The release of free copper and copper salts modifies endometrial secretions as well as cervical mucous. The hormonal IUD has a similar mechanism of action. The progestin causes the endometrium to become decidualized, resulting in atrophy of the endometrial glands. Levonorgestrel systems also generate thickened cervical mucous prohibiting sperm from penetrating this barrier [11]. All three devices allow for immediate restoration of fertility once removed.

The most common side effects include: vulvovaginitis, abdominal or pelvic pain, acne, ovarian cysts, headache, dysmenorrhea, breast pain or tenderness, intermenstrual bleeding, altered or depressed mood, menorrhagia, vaginal discharge and possible expulsion [12]. Bleeding and cramping are usually more severe within the first few months of insertion. NSAIDs can be given to reduce pain and bleeding during this time. Initiation of NSAIDs can begin at the onset of menses each month to aid in the alleviation of symptoms. Patients using the copper IUD may experience increased vaginal bleeding while patients using the levonorgestrel IUD often develop amenorrhea. With the levonorgestrel IUD, 70% of patients experience oligomenorrhea, while up to 40% experience amenorrhea within 2 years of usage [13]. It is not uncommon for women to note an increase in vaginal discharge. The physician should be diligent in performing a pelvic exam to rule out any type of cervical or vaginal infection when warranted.

Complications associated with IUDs are rare. The expulsion rate of the copper IUD within the first year is approximately 5% [14]. The risk of expulsion is higher among younger women when compared to older women. The cumulative expulsion rate for the levonorgestrel system has been 8% in nulligravid patients [15]. Expulsion is associated with bleeding, cramping, or absence of the IUD strings. Other complications include method failure, infection, and perforation. Perforation occurs in 1 per 1,000 insertions or less. Placement should be confirmed with ultrasound [16]. The incidence of pelvic inflammatory disease is only increased the first month after insertion [17]. Early IUD related infection is typically the result of endogenous cervicovaginal flora ascending into the endometrial cavity during insertion of the IUD. The organisms are usually polymicrobial or the result of a pre-existing infection. High-risk populations may be screened prior to or at the time of insertion. Prophylactic antibiotics are not recommended at time of insertion. Women suspected of having a cervicitis or infection should be treated prior to IUD placement. Although the risk is low, women with an untreated STI are more likely to develop PID after IUD placement. Women diagnosed with STI prior to insertion, in which delayed insertion was implemented, should have a negative test of cure at least 3-4 weeks prior to IUD insertion. IUDs do not prevent sexually transmitted infections. Women desiring protection from STIs should use a condom. All IUD users should have STI screening according to CDC guidelines. [18].

Aside from pregnancy prevention, IUDs also provide non-contraceptive benefit. The levonorgestrel IUD decreases dysmenorrhea and menorrhagia, often times improving related anemia [19]. Furthermore, evidence has shown it is helpful for heavy bleeding from uterine fibroids [20]. IUDs have a protective affect against endometrial hyperplasia and uterine polyps [21, 22]. They can also serve as a treatment option for pain control in patients with endometriosis [23].

The safe insertion of an intrauterine system can be accomplished at any time after delivery, spontaneous miscarriage or induced abortion, or at any time during the menstrual cycle [24]. IUD placement immediately following a vaginal delivery can be performed without an increased association of infection, uterine perforation, postpartum bleeding or uterine subinvolution. Immediate placement versus delayed insertion at 4-8 weeks postpartum is associated with an increased expulsion rate [25]. The differences in expulsion rate were the same when compared to manual insertion versus insertion with ring forceps. IUD placement at time of cesarean section may be associated with a lower expulsion rate when compared to placement following vaginal delivery [26]. Strings may not always be visualized when placed at time of cesarean. Postpartum follow up with a pelvic exam and sonogram can confirm proper placement. Immediate postpartum placement following vaginal delivery or cesarean is contraindicated in women with peripartum chorioamnionitis, endometritis, or puerperal sepsis [27].

IUDs may be placed immediately after a first trimester abortion. Women who undergo abortion services are at a greater risk for a repeat unintended pregnancy within 1 year. A single visit for this service may drastically reduce the number of unintended pregnancies [28]. In fact, 42% of women who delay insertion fail to return to follow up [29]. It is imperative to evaluate each case individually and assess when immediate insertion is warranted. For patients undergoing second trimester procedures, IUD placement is recommended after involution of the uterus. When placing an IUD at any time during the menstrual cycle, a negative pregnancy test should be confirmed. To ensure that a woman is not pregnant, insertion can be done one week following the onset of menses [30].

The copper IUD is the only intrauterine system that can be used as an emergency form of contraception. Its first reported use as such was in 1976 [31]. A fairly recent prospective cohort trial found a pregnancy rate of 0.2% when the copper IUD is inserted within 5 days of unprotected intercourse [32]. One of the greatest benefits to this form of emergency contraception is its continued use as a LARC method for these patients. Patients with a previous history of ectopic pregnancy are candidates for IUD use. The risk of future ectopic pregnancies is not increased with IUD usage. In fact, a WHO multicenter study concluded that IUD users were 50% less likely to have an ectopic pregnancy than women using no contraception [33]. The risk of ectopic pregnancy is 0.20 per 1000 women. If pregnancy does occur with IUD in place however, the risk of ectopic is greater and the pregnancy is likely to be extrauterine.

Long acting reversible contraceptive methods are the safest and most effective form of reversible contraception available. The national survey of family growth found that LARC use is higher among women aged 25-34 at 11.1%, compared to 5.0% of women aged 15-24 and 5.3% of women aged 35-44 [34]. LARC methods have an 80% continuation rate after one year. Only 55% of women who chose a non-long acting method were found to be continuing their method of choice one year after initiation of that method. Women who chose methods other than LARC were found to be 20 times more likely to have an unintended pregnancy. There are few contraindications to LARC methods. Adolescents and nulliparous women are candidates for LARC [35, 36]. The American College of Obstetricians and Gynecologists recommends that LARC be offered as the first line contraceptive method for all patients meeting eligibility criteria [37].

A careful history and physical is imperative prior to the initiation of contraception. Patient selection is important to increase satisfaction and compliance. Whether using the IUD or the implant, 3-6 month satisfaction for both remains every high. At both 3 and 6 months, 90% of women were satisfied with their LARC method. Appropriate counseling about the potential side effects not only allows patients to determine which method may be best for them, it also gives them insight into what to expect for the first few months while using that particular method [38]. Women who experience heavy bleeding, have a bleeding disorder, or are anticoagulated will not be good candidates for the copper IUD. The copper IUD is contraindicated in Wilson's disease. The IUD may not be the best choice for patients with abnormal uterine anatomy such as a uterine anomaly, submucosal myoma, or any abnormality that may disrupt the uterine cavity and interrupt proper placement or accommodation of the IUD. The IUD is suitable for patients with diabetes mellitus, obesity, sickle cell, seizure disorder, history of migraines, and hypertension [39].

Implant

The contraceptive implant is subdermally placed in the upper arm. It is small, soft, and flexible. The implant measures 4cm in length and consists of an ethylene vinyl acetate copolymer core containing 68mg of etonogestrel surrounded by an ethylene vinyl acetate copolymer skin. The ethylene vinyl acetate copolymer permits release of etonogestrel over a period of 3 years. The hormone is released at an initial rate of 67 micrograms/day decreasing to 30 micrograms/day after 2 years. The implant inhibits ovulation by altering the hypothalamic-pituitary axis. It also causes thickening of cervical mucous and modification of the endometrial lining [40, 41, and 42].

The implant is the most effective method of reversible contraception available. It has a 0.05% pregnancy rate with both typical and perfect use. Eighty four percent of women continue this form of contraception after one year [43]. The most common side effect is a change in menstrual bleeding patterns. Changes involve amenorrhea, oligomenorrhea, or prolonged bleeding. Other common side effects include: mood swings, depressed mood, weight gain, headache, acne, vaginitis, breast pain, gastrointestinal upset, dysmenorrhea, back pain, dizziness and pain at the site of insertion. Aside from menstrual irregularities, weight gain, mood swings, headache and acne are the most common side effects that lead to early discontinuation of the implant [44].

Menstrual irregularities account for a large percentage of women who seek early removal of the implant. About 20% of women report amenorrhea, while 12% report prolonged bleeding. Twenty seven percent of women report infrequent episodes of bleeding, whereas 6% report frequent episodes of bleeding [45]. Weight gain is another common concern among women using or seeking contraception. It is estimated that 6-12% of implant users report weight gain, with about 3-7% of these women discontinuing this method due to increased weight [46, 47]. Although there is limited data, current literature confirms that the implant has little to no effect on bone mineral density. Patients may report an increase in acne. Approximately 10-14% of users will experience worsening in acne symptoms, while others report an improvement in symptoms [48].

The implant can be inserted at any time of the menstrual cycle as long as pregnancy has been excluded. Insertion is recommended within five days of the last menstrual period. If not done within this timeframe, then a backup form of contraception should be utilized. The implant may be initiated after childbirth, abortion or immediately after converting to another contraceptive method [49]. The implant can be inserted immediately postpartum or 4-6 weeks after delivery in breastfeeding women. A randomized trial comparing postpartum insertion of the implant at days 1-3 postpartum compared to insertion at 4-8 weeks was conducted. The study reported no differences in breastfeeding outcomes in regard to lactogenesis and risk of lactation failure [50]. The implant can also be inserted immediately following a second or third trimester termination. The studies supporting this however, were conducted using the levonorgestrel implant system that is no longer promoted in the

United States [51]. The etonorgestrel implant can be used post abortion as well.

The insertion of the contraceptive implant usually takes five minutes. Only health care providers who receive training from the manufacturer are allowed to insert the implant. Swelling, irritation or bruising may occur at the site. About 0.2 to 1.9% of women are affected. Correct placement is confirmed by palpation. Removals can become challenging due to deep insertion, fibrosis, or migration. Removal is typically uneventful but complications do arise, and can be seen in up to 1.7% of removals [52]. Once removed, ovulation resumes quickly. Ninety percent of women ovulate within one month of removal, and 90% will resume a regular menstrual cycle with 3 months of removal [53].

As with the IUD, the implant is suitable for most candidates. Absolute contraindications include: thromboembolic disease, undiagnosed genital bleeding, acute liver disease, benign or malignant liver disease, or unknown or suspected breast cancer [54]. The implants can be a viable option for patients with the following comorbidities: dyslipidemia, diabetes mellitus, hypertension, migraine. It can also be used in patients with uterine anomalies who are not good candidates for the intrauterine system [55]. The implant is an excellent option for adolescents as well. In fact, the Choice project confirmed that among the participants, 64% chose LARC. Among these users aged 14-17, 63% of them chose the implant. Aside from its effectiveness, its appeal to this age group relied on its low maintenance requirement, improvement in acne, and relief of dysmenorrhea. The local arm insertion allows avoidance of pelvic exams, which can invoke fear and anxiety in all patients particularly young ones [56]. As with the IUD, the implant has a high satisfaction rate and most women are pleased at the six-month interval.

LARC methods provide safe contraceptive options with few exceptions. Despite numerous advantages to these methods, overall usage nationwide is low. Providers need to educate themselves as well as patients about the options available. Providers also need to dispel any misconceptions about usage and side effects. When providing sexual and reproductive services, providers and consultants need to incorporate LARC into their clinical practice and help ensure that eligible patients have access to the most effective means of pregnancy prevention.

References

[1] Jensen, Jeffry T. and Daniel R. Mishell, Jr. Family Planning. *Comprehensive Gynecology.* 6th edition. p215-16.

[2] Hathaway M, Torres L, Vollett-Krech J, Wohltjen H. Increasing LARC Utilization: Any Woman, Any Place, Any Time. *Clinical Obstetrics and Gynecology.* Volume 57. Number 4, 718-730. 2014.

[3] Deidrich J, Desai S, Zhao Q, Secura G, Madden T, Peipert J. Association of short-term bleeding and cramping patterns with long-acting reversible contraceptive method satisfaction. *American Journal of Obstetrics and Gynecology.* July 2014.

[4] Trussell, J. (2011) Contraceptive failures in the United States. *Contraception,* 397-404

[5] IUD Taskforce. http://iudtaskforce.org/IUDBasics#_edn8

[6] Sivin, I, Stern J, Coutinho E, Mattos CE, el Mahgoub S, Diaz S, Pavez M, Alvarez F, Brache V, Thevenin F, Diaz J, Faundes A, Margarita Diaz M, McCarthy T, Mishell DR, Shoupe D. (1991). Prolonged intrauterine contraception: a seven-year randomized study of the levonorgestrel 20mcg/day (LNg20) and the Copper T380 Ag IUDS. Contraception, 44(5): 473-80

[7] Trussell, J. (2011) Contraceptive failures in the United States. *Contraception,* 397-404

[8] Skyla: Official Website. http://hcp.skyla-us.com/index.php

[9] http://labeling.bayerhealthcare.com/html/products/pi/Skyla_PI.pdf

[10] Ortiz ME and Croxatto HB. (1987). The mode of action of IUDs. *Contraception.* 36(1): 37-53

[11] Long-Acting Reversible Contraception: Implants and Intrauterine Devices. The American College of Obstetricians and Gynecologists. *Practice Bulletin 121.* Reaffirmed 2013.

[12] Mirena. http://hcp.mirena-us.com/index.php

[13] Hidalgo M, Bahomondes L, Perrotti M, Diaz J, Dantas-Monteiro C, Petta C. (2002). Bleeding patterns and clinical performance of the levonorgestrel-releasing intrauterine system (Mirena) up to two years. *Contraception.* 65(2): 129-32.

[14] Rivera R, Chen-Mok M, McMullen S. (1999). Analysis of client characteristics that may affect early discontinuation of the TCu-380A IUD. *Contraception.* 60(3): 155-60.

[15] Paterson H, Ashton J, Harrison-Woolrych M. (2009). A nationwide cohort study of the use of the levonorgestrel intrauterine device in New Zealand adolescents.

[16] Long-Acting Reversible Contraception: Implants and Intrauterine Devices. The American College of Obstetricians and Gynecologists. *Practice Bulletin* 121. Reaffirmed 2013.

[17] Farley TM, Rosenberg MJ, Rowe PJ, Chen JH, Meirik O. (1992) Intrauterine devices and pelvic inflammatory disease: an international perspective. *Lancet.* 339(8796): 785-8.

[18] Long-Acting Reversible Contraception: Implants and Intrauterine Devices. The American College of Obstetricians and Gynecologists. *Practice Bulletin 121.* Reaffirmed 2013.

[19] Cihangir U, Ebru A, Murat E, Levent Y. (2013). Mechanism of action of the levonorgestrel-releasing intrauterine system in the treatment of heavy menstrual bleeding. *International Journal of Gynaecology and Obstetrics.* 123(2): 146-9.

[20] Murat Naki M, Tekcan C, Ozcan N, Cebi M. (2010). Levonorgestrel-releasing intrauterine device insertion ameliorates leiomyoma-dependent menorrhagia among women of reproductive age without a significant regression in the uterine and leiomyoma volumes. *Fertility and Sterility.* 91(1): 371-4.

[21] Lin M, Xu X, Wang Y, Hu Y, Zhao Y. (2014). Evaluation of a levonorgesterol-releasing intrauterine system for treating endometrial hyperplasia in patients with polycystic ovary syndrome. *Gynecology and Obstetric Investigation.* 78(1): 41-4.

[22] Fu Y and Zhuang Z. (2014). Long-term effects of levonorgestrel-releasing intrauterine system on tamoxifen-treated breast cancer patients: a meta-analysis. *International Journal of Clinical and Experimental Pathology.* 7(10): 6419-29.

[23] Bahamondes L, Petta CA, Fernandes A, Monteiro I. (2007). Use of the levonorgestrel-releasing intrauterine system in women with endometriosis, chronic pelvic pain and dysmenorrheal. *Contraception.* 75(6 Suppl): S134-9.

[24] Zhuang L, Wang H, Yang P. (1987). Observations of the clinical efficacies and side effects of six different timings of IUD insertions. *Clinical Journal of Obstetrics and Gynecology.* 22:350.

[25] Celen S, Moroy P, Sucak A, Aktulay A, Danisman N. (2004). Clinical outcomes of early postplacental insertion of intrauterine contraceptive devices. *Contraception.* 69(4): 279-82.

[26] Zhou S and Chi I. (1991). Immediate postpartum IUD insertions in a Chinese hospital—A two-year follow-up. *International Journal of Gynaecology and Obstetrics.* 35(2): 157-64.
[27] Long-Acting Reversible Contraception: Implants and Intrauterine Devices. *The American College of Obstetricians and Gynecologists. Practice Bulletin 121.* Reaffirmed 2013.
[28] Steenland MW, Tepper NK, Curtis KM, Kapp N. (2011) Intrauterine contraceptive insertion postabortion: a systematic review. *Contraception.* 84(5): 447-64.
[29] Gillett PG, Lee NH, Yuzpe AA, Cerskus I. (1980). A comparison of the efficacy and acceptability of the Copper-7 intrauterine device following immediate or delayed insertion after first-trimester therapeutic abortion. *Fertility and Sterility.* 34: 121-4.
[30] PB 22
[31] Lippes J, Malik T, Tatum HJ. (1976). The postcoital copper-T. *Advances in Planned Parenthood.* 11(1): 24-9.
[32] Zhou L, Xiao B. (2001). Emergency contraception with Multilo ad Cu-375 SL IUD: a multicenter clinical trial. *Contraception.* 64: 107-12.
[33] WHO Special Programme of Research, Development and Research Training in Human Reproduction, Task Force on Intrauterine Devices for Fertility Regulation, A multinational case-control study of ectopic pregnancy (1985). *Clinical Reproduction and Fertility.* 3(2): 131-43.
[34] Daniels K, Daughtery J, Jones J. Current Contraceptive Status Among Women Ages 15-44: United States, 2011-2013. NCHS Data Brief, Vol 173; December 2014. http://www.cdc.gov/nchs/data/databriefs /db173. pdf
[35] Hathaway M, Torres L, Vollett-Krech J, Wohltjen H. Increasing LARC Utilization: Any Woman, Any Place, Any Time. *Clinical Obstetrics and Gynecology.* Volume 57. Number 4, 718-730. 2014
[36] The Contraceptive Choice Project. http://www.choiceproject.wustl.edu/~ /media/Files/ChoiceProject/Study-Findings-20120917.ashx
[37] Increasing Use of Contraceptive Implants and Intrauterine Devices to Reduce Unintended Pregnancy. *The American College of Obstetricians and Gynecologists. Committee Opinion 450.* Reaffirmed 2011.
[38] Deidrich J, Desai S, Zhao Q, Secura G, Madden T, Peipert J. Association of short-term bleeding and cramping patterns with long-acting reversible contraceptive method satisfaction. *American Journal of Obstetrics and Gynecology.* July 2014.

[39] Use of Hormonal Contraception in Women With Coexisting Medical Conditions. *The American College of Obstetricians and Gynecologists. Practice Bulletin 73*. Reaffirmed 2013.

[40] Long-Acting Reversible Contraception: Implants and Intrauterine Devices. *The American College of Obstetricians and Gynecologists. Practice Bulletin 121*. Reaffirmed 2013.

[41] Speroff M, Fitz M. Clinical Gynecologic Endocrinology and Infertility. Long-acting methods of contraception. 8th edition. 2011. p1061.

[42] Nexplanon. http://www.nexplanon.com/en/consumer/about-it/what-is-nexplanon/

[43] Long-Acting Reversible Contraception: Implants and Intrauterine Devices. The American College of Obstetricians and Gynecologists. Practice Bulletin 121. Reaffirmed 2013.

[44] Nexplanon. http://www.nexplanon.com/en/consumer/about-it/what-is-nexplanon/

[45] Jensen, Jeffry T. and Daniel R. Mishell, Jr. *Family Planning. Comprehensive Gynecology*. 6th edition. p255-256.

[46] Darney P, Patel A, Rosen K, Shapiro LS, Kaunitz AM. Safety and efficacy of a single-rod etonogestrel implant (Implanon): results from 11 international clinical trials. *Fertility Sterility* 2009; 91: 1646-53.

[47] Varma R, Sinha D, Gupta JK. Non-contraceptive uses of levonorgestrel-releasing hormone system (LNG-IUS)—a systematic enquiry and overview. *Eur J Obstet Gynecol Reprod Biol* 2006; 125:9-28.

[48] Long-Acting Reversible Contraception: Implants and Intrauterine Devices. The American College of Obstetricians and Gynecologists. Practice Bulletin 121. Reaffirmed 2013.

[49] Long-Acting Reversible Contraception: Implants and Intrauterine Devices. The American College of Obstetricians and Gynecologists. Practice Bulletin 121. Reaffirmed 2013.

[50] Gurtcheff SE, Turok DK, Stoddard G, Murphy PA, Gibson M, Jones KP. Lactogenesis after early postpartum use of the contraceptive implant, *Obstet Gynecol* 2011: 117:1114-21.

[51] Long-Acting Reversible Contraception: Implants and Intrauterine Devices. The American College of Obstetricians and Gynecologists. Practice Bulletin 121. Reaffirmed 2013.

[52] A New Progestin Implant for Long-Term Contraception. *The Medial Letter. American College of Obstetricians and Gynecologists.* Vol 109, NO. 4, April 2007.

[53] Jensen, Jeffry T. and Daniel R. Mishell, Jr. Family Planning. *Comprehensive Gynecology.* 6th edition. p256.
[54] Speroff M, Fitz M. Clinical Gynecologic Endocrinology and Infertility. Long-acting methods of contraception. 8th edition. 2011. p1062.
[55] Use of Hormonal Contraception in Women With Coexisting Medical Conditions. The American College of Obstetricians and Gynecologists. Practice Bulletin 73. Reaffirmed 2013.
[56] McNicholas, C and Peipert J. Long-acting reversible contraception for adolescents. *Current Opinion.* Vol 24, Number 5. October 2012.

Sterilization

Background

Permanent sterilization is one of the oldest modern methods of fertility control that dates back to the 19th century. Couples choose sterilization when childbearing is no longer desired, when reversible methods are unattainable or inconvenient, or when projected family size is complete. Female sterilization offers an immediate form of contraception that is permanent, lifelong, and has limited side effects. The procedure typically requires no follow up on behalf of the patient outside of surgical follow up. It also places little to no demands on the sexual partner. Sterilization is often the only method of contraception for some women. In fact, up to 50% of women who undergo sterilization have never used another form of contraception prior to their procedure [1].

Over 200 million women of reproductive age worldwide use sterilization as their form of family planning. Approximately 180 million use female sterilization, and over 40 million use male sterilization with vasectomy [2]. In the United States between 2011-2013, an estimated 62% of the 60.9 million women aged 15-44 used some form of contraception. The most common form of contraception was the contraceptive pill at 16%, followed by female sterilization at 15.5%, male condoms at 9.4% and long-acting reversible contraceptives at 7.2%. Nearly one third of women aged 35-44 used female sterilization. Female sterilization is higher among older women than younger women, with less than 1% of women age 15-24 using female sterilization as contraception. Current use of female sterilization is highest among non-Hispanic black females at 21.3% compared with non-Hispanic white females at 14%. Data supports that higher educational attainment is associated with a decrease in permanent sterilization procedures [3].

Women who have decided that childbearing is complete are candidates for sterilization. These patients should fully understand the permanent nature of the procedure as well as the risk of failure, the risk of regret, and alternatives for the procedure. Patient age and parity should not impede any sterilization procedure once the patient has made a well-informed decision. A complete medical history and physical is necessary prior to sterilization surgery. The patient's medical history, health insurance coverage, compliance with follow up, ability to tolerate an office procedure and prior surgical history must be considered prior to selecting a particular sterilization procedure [4].

Sterilization Options

Female sterilization can be performed at any time. The timing of the procedure is dependent on patient preference, insurance coverage, medical assessment, and surgical approach. Surgical options include postpartum sterilization, post-abortion sterilization or interval procedures that can be done via hysteroscopy, laparoscopy, or laparotomy.

Postpartum sterilization can be done at time of cesarean or after a vaginal delivery. When the procedure is done following vaginal delivery, a minilaparatomy is generally performed via a small infraumibilical incision. The procedure is typically performed 12-24 hours after delivery to ensure that uterine involution has not occurred. The procedure can be done under general or regional anesthesia, and often the epidural placed during delivery can be left in place for the sterilization procedure. Sterilization does not require prolonged hospitalization when done postpartum [5].

Various techniques can be used to interrupt tubal patency. Commonly used methods include the Pomeroy, modified Pomeroy, and the Parkland. The Irving, Uchida, or Kroener fimbriectomy are rarely used and involve increased dissection, which often increases operative time and possible injury to the mesosalpinx. Fimbreictomy has a high failure rate as a result of recanalization of the proximal tubal segment [6, 7]. Postpartum sterilization with partial salpingectomy is the most effective method of sterilization [8].

Consent for postpartum tubal should be signed during the prenatal course. Health care providers should be familiar with states laws and hospital requirements to ensure access to the procedure postpartum. It is estimated that 46.7% of women who requested postpartum sterilization services did not receive them. The physician must advocate on behalf of their patients to ensure that sterilization is not prolonged to a later date, which in turn may result in an unwanted pregnancy [9].

Sterilization can be performed immediately following an uncomplicated spontaneous abortion or voluntary interruption of pregnancy. Following a first or second trimester termination, tubal occlusion can be performed via laparoscopy or minilaparotomy. Hysteroscopic sterilization would have to be delayed post termination [10].

When sterilization is performed outside of pregnancy, there are multiple surgical methods to be considered. Options include laparoscopy, laparotomy and hysteroscopy. Laparoscopy is performed as an outpatient procedure. The laparoscopic approach allows the provider to inspect the abdomen and pelvis, and is an immediate form of sterilization. The procedure is done under general anesthesia. Incisions are typically small and patients are quick to recover postoperatively. The disadvantages of laparoscopy include the risks associated with laparoscopic surgery including: risk of anesthesia, and risk of injury to major abdominal organs or blood vessels. Laparoscopy is generally safe and effective when used to perform sterilization. Major complications are infrequent, and account for 0.1-3.5% of procedures. Laparoscopic tubal occlusion can be achieved using electrocoagulation, mechanical devices or tubal excision [11]. Pregnancy must be ruled out prior to any sterilization procedure.

The CREST study, an investigation of more than 10,000 women undergoing tubal ligation during the period 1978-1986, documented higher failure rates than reported elsewhere in the literature. The cumulative 10 year pregnancy rate was 18.5/1000 or 1.85%. The pregnancy rate with Hulka clips was highest at 36.5/1000 or 3.65%, and lowest with unipoloar coagulation and postpartum partial salpingectomy, with failure rates of 7.5/1000 or 0.75%. The CREST study authors attribute the higher failure rates to improper techniques at the time of placement. Maintaining an adequate portion of the tube is vital for proper placement of the silicone band. Proper placement of the clips is important for maximum effectiveness. When using bipolar coagulation, it is imperative that the bipolar mode is appropriately set, and that coagulation of at least three contiguous areas of the isthmic portion of the fallopian tube is performed [12, 13].

Tubal excision with complete or partial salpingectomy may be reserved for tubal abnormality or pathology. This can be done using bipolar or monopolar technology. In light of new data suggesting that the fallopian tubes may be the origin of ovarian serous carcinoma, salpingectomy may become common practice for female sterilization.

Minilaparatomy is typically reserved for postpartum sterilization. It can also be considered for morbidly obese patients, or patients who have failed a laparoscopic approach. The same techniques for postpartum tubal ligation are generally used in this setting. In randomized trials, there was no difference in major morbidity between women who underwent tubal occlusion procedures performed by laparoscopy compared to laparotomy. When an excision method is used, tubal segments should be evaluated by pathology for confirmation [14].

Hysteroscopic sterilization offers the only outpatient procedure available for sterilization. In fact, the procedure is often performed in the office setting with local anesthesia (paracervical block) and oral or intravenous sedation. This procedure is favorable for candidates who desire a quick recovery time, want to circumvent anesthesia, and avoid surgical scars. There are two hysteroscopic methods approved for use in the United States. Adiana is one method that involves radiofrequent energy and implant placement. It is not currently available in the U.S. The other method is Essure. The Essure device was approved in 2002, and involves the transcervical insertion of a 4cm implant into each fallopian tube. The implant is comprised of a stainless steel inner coil and nickel titanium outer coil that causes an inflammatory reaction and tissue growth in response to the implantation of the device. This procedure can be done 6 weeks postpartum or post termination service [15].

Complications of hysteroscopic sterilization include the following: tubal perforation, improper placement of the coil inserts, expulsion of the occlusion devices, and other complications associated with hysteroscopy. Tubal perforation occurs in 1-3% of cases, improper placement in 0.5-3% of cases, and coil expulsion in 0.4-2.2% of cases. The most common complication is vasovagal syncope, which complicated up to 2.7% of cases. Most patients experience bleeding, and cramping during the actual placement as well as postoperatively [16].

It is important to counsel patients on the fact that Essure is not immediately permanent. Another form of contraception is needed until tubal occlusion is confirmed. Patients can be placed on OCPs or Depo Provera prior to placement of the Essure, and then continue on this method until confirmation of tubal occlusion. Confirmation of occlusion is established by hysterosalpingogram 3 months following the procedure. Compliance with postoperative HSG ranges from 13-71%. Patient selection for this procedure is important and if adherence to follow-up is a concern for the provider or patient, then another method may be preferred [17, 18]. There are no documented pregnancies reported for those women in clinical trials with tubal occlusion confirmed by HSG after bilateral placement of Essure. After successful placement, the data showed that 3.5% of women had tubal patency confirmed by HSG. Six month follow-up for these women showed 0% patency. This method is very effective when follow up of the confirmatory test is ensured [19, 20].

There are few medical contraindications to LARC contraception. LARC methods are as effective at tubal occlusion with lower morbidity and mortality. Patients who are not appropriate surgical candidates or who are ambivalent about the permanent nature of sterilization may be offered the IUD or implant for contraception.

Although women who undergo tubal occlusion are likely to report a change in bleeding patterns, the CREST study data found that women who underwent sterilization were not more likely than controlled subjects to report persistent changes in menses [21]. They were likely to report favorable changes such as a decrease in the amount of bleeding per month, a decrease in the length of flow, and a decrease in menstrual pain. The method of occlusion did not have an effect on the reported findings [22, 23].

Tubal occlusion provides some benefit outside of pregnancy prevention. Observational studies support that laparoscopic tubal occlusion reduces the risk of ovarian cancer. Tubal occlusion has a protective effect in women at high risk for ovarian cancer due to BRCA1 and BRCA2 mutations [24]. Recent data suggests that ovarian cancer may originate from the fimbria or distal portion of the fallopian tube, and its removal at time of sterilization may protect against serous ovarian carcinoma [25]. The Society of Gynecologic Oncology made a statement in December 2013 regarding salpingectomy as an "appropriate and feasible strategy for ovarian cancer reduction". For women at population risk for ovarian cancer, salpingectomy can be performed at time of hysterectomy, tubal ligation, and at the time of other pelvic surgery [26].

Tubal occlusion has also been shown to reduce the spread of organisms from the lower genital tract to the peritoneal cavity. This reduction can provide some protection against pelvic inflammatory disease. Occlusion does not provide complete protection and ascending infection leading to PID or tubo-ovarian abscess can occur in patients who have undergone tubal occlusion. It is important to always advise condom use for the prevention of STIs and HIV [27].

Women who decide to proceed with sterilization need to be 100% certain about their decision. Materials and counseling need to be provided, and patients need to be well aware that reversal of the procedure to restore fertility will require surgery, can be costly, and may not guarantee fertility without the use of reproductive assisted technology. Most women do not regret their decision. A prospective analysis of CREST data found that the cumulative regret rate over 14 years was 12.7% [28]. The risk of regret is higher for women who have the procedure performed at 30 years of age or younger. The risk of regret for women over 30 is 5.8% compared to 20.3% of women aged 30 and younger [29]. Women age 30 and younger were 3-38 times more likely to regret having the procedure. Patients who underwent post-abortive sterilization did not have an associated increased risk in regret. The risk of regret is reduced with proper counseling and a comprehensive discussion of associated risks [30].

Male Sterilization

When counseling female patients on sterilization options, it is appropriate to include vasectomy as a viable option for her partner. Vasectomy is safer than tubal occlusion. This outpatient procedure has a rapid recovery and is often times less costly than tubal occlusion [31]. Complications following the procedure are rather uncommon with less than 3% requiring medical attention [32]. Vasectomy is the most common urologic procedure, and is used by nearly 7% of married couples as the sole form of contraception. There has been a range of techniques developed to occlude the vas deferens. These techniques include excision and ligation, surgical clips, thermal and electrocautery, and chemical occlusion. The no-scalpel vasectomy has become the technique of choice amongst surgeons in North America. Compared with other techniques, this method reduces the incision size, procedure time, pain, bleeding, and postoperative complications [33]. Minor complications resulting from vasectomy include: infection at the site of the incision, bleeding, hematoma formation, granuloma formation, and epididymitis. These complications occur in 0.4-10% of cases [34, 35]. There is no increased risk of impotence, and sexual function is not affected [36]. Vasectomy is not immediately effective and will require another form of contraception until semen analysis confirms azoospermia. Although most men are azoospermic three months after the procedure, 98-99% of patients will achieve azoospermia by 6 months post operatively [37].

Deciding to put an end to one's fertility can be a difficult decision. The decision making process requires ample time to weigh the advantages and disadvantages of all options available. Providers should facilitate this process and provide adequate counseling and resources to ensure that patients make an informed decision that is individualized, safe and effective. Although women seek family planning services through Obstetric and Gynecologic consultation, it is critical that providers discuss all reasonable options, including vasectomy. Women have the right to plan their families accordingly, and services to aid in this should be provided in a comprehensive, informative, and unprejudiced manner.

References

[1] EngenderHealth. Contraceptive Sterilization: Global Issues and Trends. http://www.cdc.gov/nchs/data/databriefs/db173.pdf

[2] EngenderHealth. Contraceptive Sterilization: Global Issues and Trends. http://www.cdc.gov/nchs/data/databriefs/db173.pdf

[3] Daniels K, Daughtery J, Jones J. Current Contraceptive Status Among Women Ages 15-44: United States, 2011-2013. NCHS Data Brief, Vol 173; December 2014. http://www.cdc.gov/nchs/data/databriefs/ db173. pdf

[4] Benefits and Risks of Sterilization. American College of Obstetricians and Gynecologists. *Practice Bulletin,* Number 133. February 2013.

[5] Berghella V, Landon M. Cesarean Delivery. Gabbe Obstetrics: Normal and Problem Pregnancies. P472-476.

[6] Sterilization. Williams Obstetrics. Ch 39.

[7] Pati S, Cullins V. Female sterilization: evidence. *Obstet Gynecol Clin North Am* 27:859, 2000.

[8] Peterson HB, Xia Z, Hughes JM, Wilcomx LS, Tylor LR, Trussels J. The Risk of Pregnancy After Tubal Sterilization: Findings From the U.S. Collaborative Review of Sterilization. *Am J Obstet Gynecol* 1996: 174:1161-8.

[9] Thurman AR, Janecek T. One-year follow-up of women with unfulfilled postpartum sterilization requests. *Obstet Gynecol* 2010; 116: 1071-7.

[10] Benefits and Risks of Sterilization. American College of Obstetricians and Gynecologists. *Practice Bulletin,* Number 133. February 2013.

[11] Benefits and Risks of Sterilization. American College of Obstetricians and Gynecologists. *Practice Bulletin*, Number 133. February 2013.

[12] Peterson HB, Xia Z, Hughes JM, Wilcomx LS, Tylor LR, Trussels J. The Risk of Pregnancy After Tubal Sterilization: Findings From the U.S. Collaborative Review of Sterilization. *Am J Obstet Gynecol* 1996: 174:1161-8.

[13] Benefits and Risks of Sterilization. American College of Obstetricians and Gynecologists. *Practice Bulletin,* Number 133. February 2013.

[14] Kulier R, Boulvain M, Walker DM, De Condolle G, Campana A. Minilaparotomy and endoscopic techniques for tubal sterilization. *Cochrane Database of Systematic Reviews* 2004, Issue3.

[15] Benefits and Risks of Sterilization. American College of Obstetricians and Gynecologists. *Practice Bulletin*, Number 133. February 2013.

[16] Benefits and Risks of Sterilization. American College of Obstetricians and Gynecologists. *Practice Bulletin,* Number 133. February 2013.

[17] Guiahi M, Goldman KN, McElhinney MM, Olson CG. Improving hysterosalpingogram confirmatory test follow-up after Essure hysteroscopic sterilization. *Contraception* 2010; 81: 520-4.

[18] Shavell VI, Abdallah ME, Diamond MP, Kmak DC, Berman JM. Post-Essure hysterosalpingography compliance in a clinic population. *J Minim Invasive Gynecol* 2008; 15:431-4.

[19] Cooper JM, Carignan CS, Cher D, Kerin JF. Microinsert nonincisional hysteroscopic sterilization. Selective Tubal Occlusion Procedure 2000 Investigators Group. *Obstet Gynecol* 2003; 102: 59-67.

[20] Kerin JF, Cooper JM, Price T, Herendeal BJ, Cayuela-Font E, Cher D, et al. Hysteroscopic sterilization using a microinsert device: results of a multicenter Phase II study. *Hum Reprod* 2003; 18: 1223-30.

[21] Peterson HB, Jeng G, Folger SG, Hillis SA, Marchbanks PA, Wilcox LS. The risk of menstrual abdnormalitis after tubal sterilization. US Collaborative Review of Sterilization Working Group. *N Engl J Med* 2000; 343:1681-7.

[22] Sinha D, Kalathy V, Gupta JK, Clark TJ. The feasibility, success and patient satisfaction associated with outpatient hysteroscopic sterilization. *BJOG.* 2007 Jun: 114 (6):676-83.

[23] Mino M, Arjona JE, Cordon J, Pelegrin B, Povedano B, Chacon E. Success rate and patient satisfaction with the Essure sterilization in an outpatient setting: a prospective study of 857 women. *BJOG* 2007: 114:763-6.

[24] Narod SA, Sun P, Ghadirian P, Lynch H, Isaacs C, Garber J, et al. Tubal ligation and risk of ovarian cancer in carriers of BRCA1 and BRCA2 mutations: a case-control study. *Lancet* 2001;357:1467-70.

[25] Benefits and Risks of Sterilization. American College of Obstetricians and Gynecologists. *Practice Bulletin,* Number 133. February 2013.

[26] Society of Gynecologic Oncology. SGO Clinical Practice Statement: Salpingectomy for Ovarian Cancer Prevention. December 2013.

https://www.sgo.org/clinical-practice/guidelines/sgo-clinical-practice-statement-salpingectomy-for-ovarian-cancer-prevention/

[27] Benefits and Risks of Sterilization. American College of Obstetricians and Gynecologists. *Practice Bulletin*, Number 133. February 2013.

[28] Hillis SD, Marchbanks PA, Tylor LR, Peterson HB. Poststerilization regret: findings from the United States Collaborative Review of Sterilization. *Obstet Gynecol* 1999; 93: 889-95.

[29] Curtis KM, Mohllajee AP, Peterson HB. Regret following female sterilization at a young age: a systematic review. *Contraception* 2006; 73:205-10.

[30] Benefits and Risks of Sterilization. American College of Obstetricians and Gynecologists. *Practice Bulletin*, Number 133. February 2013.

[31] Benefits and Risks of Sterilization. American College of Obstetricians and Gynecologists. *Practice Bulletin,* Number 133. February 2013.

[32] Cook LA, Van Vliet HAAM, Lopez LM, Pun A, Gallo MF. Vasectomy occlusion techniques for male sterilization (Review). *The Cochrane Collaboration.* 2011.

[33] White MA, Maatman TJ. Comparative Analysis of Effectiveness of Two Local Anesthetic Techniques in Men Undergoing No-Scalpel Vasectomy. *Urology* 2007 Dec;70(6):1187-9.

[34] Nirapathpongporn A, Huber DH, Krieger JN. No-scalpel vasectomy at the King's birthday vasectomy festival. *Lancet* 1009; 335:894-5.

[35] Alderman PM. Complications in a series of 1224 vasectomies. *J Fam Pract* 1991; 33:579-84.

[36] Benefits and Risks of Sterilization. American College of Obstetricians and Gynecologists. *Practice Bulletin,* Number 133. February 2013.

[37] Badrakumar C, Gogoi NK, Sundaram SK. Semem analysis after vasectomy: when and how many? *BJU Int* 2000; 86:479-81.

In: Contraception
Editor: Alicia Y. Armstrong
ISBN: 978-1-63482-145-2

Chapter 3

Contraception: New Technologies

Nicole Banks, MD and Diana Blithe ,PhD
Eunice Kennedy Shriver National Institute of Child Health and Human Development, National Institutes of Health, Bethesda, MD, US

Abstract

Despite significant improvements in contraceptive options, there continues to be a high rate of unplanned pregnancy. About half of these pregnancies occur in contraceptive users, largely due to inconsistent or incorrect use. This fact points to a significant unmet need for effective and reliable male and female contraception. Development of new contraceptive options for women is focused on meeting the following goals: decreasing the risks of current hormonal contraception and improving compliance with easier to use methods such as a transdermal patch, vaginal ring or long-acting reversible contraception options. New programs are needed to explore non-hormonal methods targeting molecules involved in ovulation, fertilization and implantation, and to identify options that have additional health benefits, such as prevention of sexually transmitted disease. Current male contraception options are limited to condoms and vasectomy; however, studies demonstrate that male hormonal contraception could be an effective option for the future. Additional research into non-hormonal approaches to testicular or epididymal targets necessary for sperm production or function may result in effective products for male contraception. Future contraceptive research and development should continue to address the above listed goals, as well as expand access to reliable contraception both within the United States and globally.

Introduction

Introduction of the oral contraceptive pill in 1960 revolutionized women's health and for the first time provided a reliable and reversible method of contraception that was controlled exclusively by women [1]. Despite significant improvements in contraceptive technologies, detailed in the second chapter of this book, current contraceptive options are failing to meet the needs of many reproductive-age women. In 2012 alone, 85 million pregnancies worldwide were unintended [2-4]. Within the United States, approximately half of all pregnancies are unintended. Mississippi and Delaware have the highest unintended pregnancy rates at 65 and 60% respectively [3]. Approximately 50% of unintended pregnancies end in abortion [4]. Half of all unintended pregnancies are in contraceptive users, primarily due to inconsistent or incorrect use of the chosen method [5, 6]. The 2002 National Survey of Family Growth showed no improvement in contraceptive effectiveness between 1995 and 2002 and, in the population of contraceptive users, the probability of failure was 12.4% by the end of one year of method use [7].

These data, as well as continued world population growth, reveal a serious unmet need for effective, reversible and easily accessible contraceptive methods [8]. There are numerous opportunities for potential improvement over the status quo. Affordability and accessibility need to be addressed both globally and within the United States. Improved long-acting systems with acceptable side effect profiles have the potential of addressing contraceptive failure resulting from inconsistent or improper use. For individuals who are not sexually active on a regular basis, effective on-demand methods would offer an alternative to longer-acting methods that may include side effects such as irregular bleeding or amenorrhea. However, coitally-dependent methods are inherently much less effective than long-acting methods and would have less impact on unplanned pregnancy rates. Development of new methods could consider strategies to provide added health benefits, such as dual protection against both pregnancy and sexually transmitted infections (STI), particularly HIV [8]. As research advances our understanding of genes, proteins and enzymes critical for reproduction, potential exists to develop new targeted methods that would decrease or eliminate systemic side effects [8]. The development of male contraceptive options has long been a goal of the scientific and family planning community; however, condoms and vasectomy are the only options currently available. Commercial investment in development of male contraception has waned despite promising advances in male hormonal contraceptive research. The reasons for diminished interest are unclear, although there is speculation that it is due to the belief that agents would not be accepted or used [9-12]; to the contrary, available data show that attitudes towards hormonal male fertility control are generally positive in much of the world [11]. In a randomized controlled trial of a transdermal gel-based male hormonal contraceptive, 56% (44/79) of men were satisfied or extremely satisfied with the studied method [10]. As commercial investment in contraceptive research for both men and women has waned, much of the work in the United States has been conducted by the *Eunice Kennedy Shriver* National Institute of Child Health and Human Development (NICHD) through a variety of programs including research grants to identify new targets/ products as well as clinical studies in its Contraceptive Clinical Trial Network (CCTN) [13].

Female Hormonal Contraception

The combined oral contraceptive (COC) pill ("the pill") revolutionized female reproductive health and is the most popular form of birth control in the United States, used by 10.5 million women [14]. Nearly all available formulations of COCs contain synthetic estrogen, ethinyl estradiol (EE), and a progestin. The major mechanism of action is to use a high dose of progestin to inhibit ovulation. The addition of EE helps to potentiate the action of the progestin and also stabilizes the endometrium to produce regular bleeding patterns when the product is used cyclically (with a short hormone-free interval at the end of each monthly supply). Comparative potency of various estrogen bioassays indicate that EE is 30-600 times more potent than natural estrogens (estradiol, estrone, estriol), and it is not effectively metabolized in the liver [13, 15, 16]. One of the most serious complications associated with use of the COC pills are vascular events related to the prothrombotic effects of EE [13, 17-19]. This risk has principally been managed by lowering the dose of EE to below 50 mcg. Most COC pills currently on the market contain 20-35 mcg EE. More recently, efforts have focused on using a different form of estrogen, such as natural estradiol, which may have an improved safety profile over EE [13]. Natazia, a new COC with estradiol valerate and the progestin, dienogest, was recently approved by the U.S. FDA. This pill has been shown to have an improved bleeding profile compared to other COCs with EE and levonorgestrel [20]. Compared with placebo, the estradiol valerate and dienogest regimen had a 67% reduction in bleeding in women with heavy menstrual bleeding, resulting in approval of the product for treatment of menorrhagia [21]. A second pill containing natural 17β estradiol and nomegestrol acetate as the progestin is approved for use in Europe but not the U.S. It has been shown to achieve effective ovulation inhibition, comparable to other pills on the market [22, 23]. Additionally, a phase IIA clinical trial of Estetrol (E4) combined with desogestrel has shown promise, with its lower potency relative to EE predicted to correlate with fewer side effects [24].

An alternative strategy for reducing the venous thrombosis risk of hormonal contraception is to use estrogen-free contraceptive options. High doses of progestins in the follicular phase will effectively inhibit ovulation. Lower doses of progestins may permit ovulation but may act by other mechanisms such as cervical mucus effects or interference with sperm function. Progesterone receptor ligands hold the potential of providing oral hormonal contraception without the side effects of estrogen. This family of medications includes progestin-only pills (POP or mini-pill), progesterone receptor antagonists, and progesterone receptor modulators (PRM), which have tissue selective agonist-antagonist properties [25]. The prototypical and most promising PRM is ulipristal acetate (UPA), a 19-norprogesterone derivative that acts as an antagonist in the ovary to inhibit ovulation but may have protective effects on breast tissue [26]. A single 30 mg dose of UPA, marketed as ella® in the United States, is approved as an emergency contraceptive by the FDA and has been shown to suppress follicular rupture for five days, even when administered in the advanced follicular phase [27, 28]. A lower dose of UPA (marketed in Europe as Esmya), used continuously for up to 6 months, has been shown to be highly effective against the pain and heavy bleeding associated with uterine fibroids. Studies are ongoing to determine whether low dose UPA may work as an alternative to the mini-pill with an improved bleeding profile [29]. Interestingly, continuous use of PRMs appears to cause endometrial anti-proliferative effects and previously undescribed changes in endometrial pathology [30, 31]. These changes are not consistent with malignancy or premalignant lesions, and have been termed PRM-associated endometrial changes (PAEC) [32]. Additional study is needed to determine the long-term consequences of these changes [32].

Alternative delivery methods of hormonal contraception are already available commercially in the form of depot injections, implants, a patch and a vaginal ring. Newer hormonal agents and combinations are being tested in non-oral forms, particularly vaginal rings and transdermal methods. A new combined EE and gestodene patch with equivalent hormonal exposure as a 20 mcg EE and 60 mcg gestodene COC showed effective ovulation inhibition and reversibility in phase III open-label multicenter trials [33]. Another patch containing levonorgestrel and EE is also in development. Additionally, a progestin-only patch using levonorgestrel is currently in phase II trials in the NICHD CCTN [13]. Nestorone, derived from 19-norprogesterone, is a highly potent non-androgenic progestin without oral bioactivity [34]. A vaginal ring with Nestorone and EE was developed and is undergoing phase III clinical trials through the International Committee for Contraceptive Research and the CCTN [13, 35]. Other Nestorone formulations currently under development include a transdermal gel and a Metered Dose Transdermal System spray [36, 37]. UPA, in addition to its clinical use discussed above, has also been studied in a contraceptive vaginal ring, with ovulation suppression in 86.1% of treatment cycles with a 2500 μg/day dose [38, 39]. PAEC was observed in 78.8% of study participants and a heavy vaginal bleeding episode occurred in 8 of 55 subjects after 6 months of continuous use [39].

Implants and injections offer contraceptive users highly reliable hormonal birth control with fewer compliance issues. Implants releasing either etonogestrel or levonorgestrel are the most effective reversible methods available for women and the typical effectiveness rates are identical with perfect use rates (99.9%) [40]. Nestorone was developed and tested as a rod implant in breastfeeding women, where it was found to be highly efficacious and safe for breastfeeding due to the lack of bioactivity when ingested by the infant [40].

The Nestorone implant was also studied as a rod implant in reproductive aged women and efficacy was acceptable, but not as effective as during the post-partum period [41]. The NICHD and WHO have investigated a new injectable contraceptive with levonorgestrel butanoate, which was effective for up to 5-6 months with a single 50 mg dose [42]. This formulation may have fewer side effects than the currently available Depot Provera injectable contraception [13].

Female Non-Hormonal Contraception

Hormonally based methods have been the cornerstone of currently available contraception; however, non-hormonal options have the potential of minimizing side effects by more specifically targeting ovulation and fertilization. Studies have shown that cyclooxygenase-2 (cox-2) inhibitors given in the late follicular phase delay follicular rupture, likely because cox-2 is an integral component of prostaglandin synthesis, which plays an important role in follicular rupture [43]. Rofecoxib, given for nine consecutive days after the dominant follicle reached 14-16 mm showed delayed follicle rupture in 4 of the 6 women who received it, compared to 0 of the 7 women who received placebo [44]. Similarly, in a separate study, 15 mg of meloxicam was given with levonorgestrel when the leading follicle was 15-17 mm and when it was greater than or equal to 18 mm. Follicular rupture or ovulatory dysfunction occurred more frequently in the group who received the meloxicam with the levonorgestrel (66% vs 88%, $P < 0.012$) [43]. Meloxicam was also tested independently by giving 15 mg/day and 30 mg/day for 5 consecutive days in the late follicular phase. Dysfunctional ovulation was seen in 90.9% of cycles with 30 mg/day [45]. The evidence surrounding cox-2 inhibitors merits further investigation of the mechanism by which this pathway can regulate ovulatory function. Other novel approaches targeting genes and proteins involved in ovulation and fertilization have proven intriguing. Phosphodiesterase 3A is expressed in mouse oocytes and has been shown to be critical for oocyte maturation and meiotic progression [46]. A phosphodiesterase 3 inhibitor, ORG 9935, tested in female macaques appeared efficacious as no animals became pregnant at serum concentrations > 300 nmol/L; this observed effect was reversible after discontinuation of the medication [47]. Future contraceptive strategies may be able to target oocyte-specific genes and their protein products that are essential for meiosis control, ovulation, fertilization, and transition from oocyte to embryo. Examples of these targets studied in animal orthologs are Wee2, Erk1/2, Juno, and Zar1, respectively [48-51]. Additional targets may develop from existing basic science research on endometrial readiness for implantation. Leukemic inhibitory factor (LIF) is one of many molecules involved in the pre-implantation window of the endometrium. A mouse model has shown that injection of a PEGylated antagonist of LIF in female mice successfully prevents implantation by acting on endometrial cells [52]. Vascular endothelial growth factor (VEGF) also plays an important role in implantation. In a mouse model and the rhesus monkey, inhibition of VEGF-A prevents implantation. Using microarray, 20 transcripts have been shown to be modified by VEGF-A inhibition and this target could represent new avenues of research for endometrium specific contraceptive development [1, 53]

Female Devices

Long-Acting Reversible Contraceptive (LARC) methods (IUDs and implants) are by far the most effective methods of contraception available to women today. The typical failure rate is 0.1, 0.2 and 0.8% for Implanon® or Jadelle®, Mirena® IUS and the ParaGard® Copper IUD, respectively, making LARCs 10-80 times more effective than the typical failure rate for COC pills, vaginal rings or patch methods [54]. The Copper IUD is also nearly 100% percent effective as emergency contraception when used within 5 days of unprotected intercourse and it has the added benefit of providing a highly effective long-term contraceptive method for the user [55]. As more women continue to accept the intrauterine device as a viable contraceptive option, development of IUSs with improved side-effect profiles would be beneficial. Currently, two low dose levonorgestrel IUSs are in clinical development. (LNG-IUS12 and LNG-IUS16) and have completed phase II clinical trials showing that they are effective and may be easier to insert than the currently available Mirena®, particularly in nulliparous women [56]. A phase II clinical trial of three etonogestrel-releasing IUSs was completed in July 2011, but results have not yet been published [57]. UPA, the PRM discussed above, was tested with an IUS in a rhesus macaque model, resulting in endometrial atrophy and amenorrhea [58]. Additionally, several progesterone receptor antagonists have been tested using an IUS in both animal models and women, and generally have produced an antiproliferative effect that may prove to have therapeutic and contraceptive uses [30, 59-61].

Male Hormonal Contraception

Current options for male contraception are condoms, which have a typical failure rate of 18% [54], and vasectomy, which lacks reversibility. Greater than 50% of men purport to be interested in alternative methods of male contraception, highlighting a significant unmet need [11, 62]. The efficacy of male hormonal contraception has been established [62-70]; however, there is no male equivalent of "the pill" available. Because men do not face the medical risks associated with pregnancy, any drug that will be used in healthy individuals for an extended period of time has particularly high expectations for safety and lack of side effects [71].

Hormonal methods are based on the knowledge that very high intra-testicular testosterone levels are required to support spermatogenesis and these intra-testicular levels can be suppressed through feedback inhibition on the hypothalamic-pituitary axis [72]. Exogenous androgens, alone or in combination with a progestin or gonadotropin-releasing hormone antagonist, feedback to the hypothalamus and pituitary and inhibit secretion of hormones, in particular LH, that stimulate local production of testosterone in the testes. Numerous studies using this approach have shown high rates of oligospermia (<3 million/mL), severe oligozoospermia (<1 million/mL) or azoospermia (no sperm) resulting in high contraceptive efficacy and good reversibility with minimal short-term side effects [62-70]. Performance is influenced by ethnicity, with apparent increased efficacy in east-Asian populations as compared to Caucasians; however, this difference is eliminated by the addition of a progestin [73, 74].

One reason that there is not a pill for male contraception is that oral testosterone is cleared too rapidly to be effective as a single daily dose regimen even in combination with a progestin. Multiple doses of oral testosterone per day would be impractical for contraception [75]. Methyltestosterone has better oral bioavailability but caused hepatotoxicity with long-term use [76]. A newly developed androgen, dimethandrolone, is a potent androgen with progestational activity [77]. Dimethandrolone undecanoate (DMAU) is a pro-drug of dimethandrolone and has potential as a single agent oral contraceptive. A phase I trial of DMAU showed that the drug was well tolerated and had improved pharmacokinetics when given with a high-fat meal [78].

The synthetic androgen, 7 alpha-methyl-19-nortestosterone (MENT), is currently being evaluated as a possible male contraception that may offer a favorable side-effect profile due to its resistance to peripheral conversion to dihydrotestosterone (DHT) by 5-alpha reductase [71, 79, 80]. MENT is more potent than testosterone and may provide selective sparing of the prostate while supporting other androgen-dependent functions [71, 80, 81]. Initial evaluations of MENT implants for use as an anti-spermatogenic agent were comparable to initial studies with testosterone, with about two-thirds of men showing dose-dependent spermatogenesis suppression [81]. Studies of MENT implants in combination with a progestin showed initial promising results but were ultimately disappointing due to declining MENT release from the implants over time [82, 83]. Improvements of the MENT implant resulting in sustained levels of MENT release require further testing in clinical trials [83].

Due to the poor oral bioavailability of testosterone, many male hormonal contraceptive studies have used a transdermal delivery method for testosterone. Transdermal testosterone gel is already clinically available to treat hypoandrogenism. One study used testosterone gel and depo-medroxyprogesterone acetate (DMPA), an injectable progestin approved for female contraception, and showed that 90% of subjects became severely oligozoospermic [84]. Notably, this method used two FDA approved products, albeit for an off-label indication. Another regimen in development used daily applications of Nestorone (NES) gel and testosterone gel (T gel) compared with T gel alone in a randomized controlled trial. The use of both NES gel (8 mg) and T gel suppressed sperm concentration to <1 million/mL or azoospermia in 89% of men compared to only 23% when testosterone gel was given alone [85, 86]. Use of a higher dose of NES (12 mg) did not improve the suppressive effects over those observed with the 8 mg dose. Using a combination of NES and T gel reduces serum gonadotropin (LH and FSH) rapidly. Gonadotropin hormone concentrations greater than 1 IU/L after 4 weeks of treatment predicted treatment failure (sperm concentration >1 million/mL) with 97% sensitivity [72]. It is unclear if failure was due to inconsistent use of the products or to non-response to the drug regimen. Study participants were surveyed on acceptability of the contraceptive regimen and over half of participants reported being satisfied or extremely satisfied with this method of contraception [10]. The results support the prospect that this regimen could be developed as a user-controlled effective method of male contraception.

Testosterone undecanoate (TU) is a long-acting ester of testosterone and has been used in a number of studies, either alone or in combination with long-acting injectable progestins or progestin implants. TU, given in monthly injections in a Chinese population, showed a high rate (>95%) of spermatogenesis suppression [87]. Men who achieved suppression (n=855) participated in a contraceptive efficacy study. In the couples who used the method for pregnancy prevention over a 2 year period, the failure rate was 1.3% [88]. TU and two doses of etonogestrel implants were studied in a double-blind, placebo controlled trial with 354 healthy male participants. Suppression of sperm counts to <l million/mL at week 16 of treatment occurred in 89% of men overall, and 94% of men who received high-release etonogestrel implants. The authors concluded that the combination could be

used as a well-tolerated male hormonal contraception, but that room for improvement remained [89, 90]. Injections of TU and norethisterone enanthate showed promise in small clinical trials [91, 92]; however, a larger trial was halted in 2011 due to the concern that side effects and risks were outweighing the potential benefits for study participants [93].

Taken together, male hormonal contraception has been extensively studied, with proven efficacy and, for the most part, an acceptable side-effect profile. It is currently the closest to becoming a commercially available product for men and many of the formulations are available as FDA-approved medications for use to treat other conditions. However, further industry interest may be needed before the dream of a male equivalent of "the pill" becomes readily available.

Male Non-Hormonal Contraception

Compared to male hormonal contraception, research into non-hormonal options is at an earlier stage of development with few phase I or II clinical trials. There remains significant untapped potential, as this area of research is rich in basic science and diversity of ideas and may produce a contraceptive with a more targeted effect and presumably few side effects. A number of pharmacologic compounds have been identified as candidates for possible male contraceptive purposes; however, some were abandoned due to toxicity and/or irreversibility [62]. One such compound, Gossypol, a polyphenolic drug isolated from cotton plants, was used in over 8000 Chinese men in the 1970s; however, the product was abandoned due to non-reversibility in some subjects and potential for side effects. Some efforts aimed at investigating the drug's use for non-surgical sterilization have continued [94, 95].

Another novel approach targets the Sertoli-germ cell junction, which, if disrupted, leads to separation of the germ cell from the seminiferous epithelium and release of immature spermatids, resulting in male infertility [96]. Indenopyridines have been shown in multiple animal studies to inhibit sperm production [97, 98]. The contraceptive effect is reversible in most tested species, but was irreversible in rat, possibly due to a higher affinity of the compound to rat Sertoli cells [98]. Testing of the indenopyridine, CDB-4022, in adult male cynomolgus monkeys showed promising results with rapid decrease in sperm concentration and full reversibility [98]. Indazole carboxylic acid derivatives (lonidamine, adjudin and H2-gamendazole) have been identified and studied in animal models [96, 99-102]. Administration of low doses of these drugs to adult male rats resulted in fully reversible infertility with no apparent effects on the hypothalamic-pituitary-testicular axis [96]. Reversibility was dose and species dependent. Adjudin primarily targets tight junctions. Specificity for the testis germ cell-Sertoli cell anchoring junction can be improved by conjugating Adjudin to a modified recombinant FSH ligand, which can serve as a 'carrier' to testicular FSH receptors, potentially reducing off-target toxicity [99-101]. H2-gamendazole at higher doses has the potential to be irreversible but lower chronic doses may improve reversibility (personal communication).

Retinoic acid (RA) is critical to initiation of meiosis, and thus, spermatogenesis. It is needed to induce expression of *Stra8*, a vertebrate specific gene responsible for meiotic initiation in both spermatogenesis and oogenesis [103, 104]. Several approaches have validated this pathway as a promising target for non-hormonal male contraception. Bisdichloro–acetyldiamines (BDADs) were long ago discovered to suppress spermatogenesis [105, 106]. One BDAD, WIN 18,446, caused infertility in murine and rabbit models, with full fertility recovery after discontinuation of the medication [104-109]. The drug was used to treat over 60 men for one year. It was well tolerated and caused excellent inhibition of spermatogenesis. However, use with alcohol caused a severe disulfiram reaction and the development of the drug was abandoned. More recently, the action of BDADS was discovered to block testicular RA biosynthesis through irreversible inhibition of alcohol dehydrogenase 1A2 [105-108]. Additional research to understand the RA pathway may lead to more specificity for the testicular effects. Studies using BMS-189453, a pan-retinoic acid receptor antagonist, also demonstrated reversible inhibition of spermatogenesis in a murine model [110]. However, higher doses in rat and rabbit models showed significant testicular toxicity and some systemic toxicity at all tested doses, limiting future therapeutic uses of the pan retinoic acid receptor antagonist [110, 111]. The retinoic acid receptor α variant is essential for spermatogenesis; thus, it is possible that more specific inhibitors can be developed that would inhibit sperm production but not exhibit systemic toxicity [112].

BRDT is a testis-specific protein that is critical for chromatin remodeling during spermatogenesis [113, 114]. Single nucleotide polymorphisms in *BRDT* were associated with oligozoospermia and azoospermia in a recent genome-wide association study [115]. Mice with homozygous *Brdt* mutations generated by targeted mutagenesis were viable but the male animals were sterile [113]. The small-molecule inhibitor, JQ1, was shown to bind to BRDT and prevent recognition of acetylated histone, H4, thus interrupting chromatin remodeling [116]. When given to male mice, JQ1 led to infertility that was completely reversible, meriting further study as a potential male contraceptive drug [116].

Calcium plays a major role in sperm motility. CatSper and KSper are sperm-specific ion channels for sperm tail calcium entry and both are required for male fertility. Gene mutations and deletions in animal models affect male fertility without apparent systemic effects [117-120]. Because of this specificity, CatSper is an appealing target for male contraception; however, little research has explored potential CatSper blockers [62]. The compound, HC-056456, may represent a potential candidate, with initial promising *in vitro* studies showing that the drug prevents hyperactivated motility of sperm, a necessary step in fertilization [121]. Progesterone activates CatSper through a non-classical progesterone binding domain and causes sperm tail hyperactivation. Physiologically, the likely source of progesterone is the cumulus oocyte complex after it enters the oviduct. Sperm bind to the wall of the oviduct and undergo capacitation [122]. They can remain viable for several days until progesterone and other signals cause them to detach, become hyperactivated, and swim toward the ampulla of the oviduct where fertilization can occur. Disruption of the interaction of progesterone with sperm targets may be another target for contraception either in men or women. This disruption of communication may be one of the mechanisms of action of drugs used for emergency contraception [Ko et al.]. Na+/H+ exchanger ion channels are also found to be important in sperm motility [123, 124]. Knock-out of the sperm-specific Na+/H+ exchanger (sNHE) gene in mice caused infertility, making this channel another potential sperm-specific target for male contraception. The Na+/K+- ATPase (sodium pump) is also known to play an important role in sperm motility and capacitation and is composed of α and β subunits [125-130]. The α4 subunit appears to be specific to the male reproductive tract [131]. Cardenolide analogues are known to inhibit Na+/K+ pumps and have been used clinically to treat congestive heart failure [132]. Ouabain, a cardenolide analog, has higher affinity for the α4 subunit than other sodium pump subunits in both mice and humans, which suggests the potential of developing ouabain derivatives with high enough specificity to be used as a male contraceptive [133].

Further advances in the understanding of sperm motility and activation continue to suggest potential future targets for male contraception development. Much of this research has centered on the integral role of protein kinases in these pathways. An early example of such work is Nomura and Vacquier's study of sea urchin sperm flagella, in which protein kinase A-dependent phosphorylation was highlighted as a critical element in flagellar motility [134]. Sperm capacitation and the acrosome reaction have also been noted to rely on protein kinases and tyrosine kinases such as the Src family [135, 136]. The significance of these pathways was detailed in a paper by Kwon, et al. in which vasopressin was noted to down-regulate protein kinase A activity in mice spermatozoa with attendant impact on sperm motility and capacitation status [137]. Protein kinases play a key role in several aspects of spermatozoa development, activation, and motility, making these proteins compelling molecular targets for male contraception; however, development of effective treatments has been hampered by lack of specificity of the available kinases, resulting in effects on unrelated molecular pathways [138]. While research in the area of protein kinases has advanced understanding of processes critical to male fertility, viable contraceptive drugs targeting these pathways have yet to be identified.

Male Devices

As an alternative to surgical vasectomy and the challenge of vasectomy reversal, research has long sought other methods for blocking the vas deferens with higher rates of reversibility or for a non-surgical vasectomy procedure [139]. In 2003, a phase II randomized controlled trial of 288 patients was conducted in China comparing an intra-vas device (IVD) to no-scalpel vasectomy [140]. The IVD is composed of a shell of urethane filled with nylon thread that allows for fluid, but not sperm to pass through the device. It is inserted using a minor procedure similar to performance of a vasectomy. The trial showed that by 12 months post-op, contraceptive success rates, based on semen analyses results, were 94.3% and 98.6% in the IVD and vasectomy groups, respectively ($p=0.054$). There was a higher satisfaction rate and fewer complications were observed in the men who received the IVD compared to the group who had no-scalpel vasectomy [140]. A different IVD in development is composed of a cross-linked composite of polyvinyl alcohol and nano-particles of silicon dioxide and copper chloride. The complex/polymer composite material has micropores designed to allow passage of fluid, but not sperm. Tested in dogs and rabbits, the IVD showed high efficacy with no pathological evidence of damage to the testes, epididymis, or vas [141, 142]. Reversibility was tested in rabbits, with pregnancy rates of 60% in the reversal group compared to 80% in a control sham-operation group. The authors suggest that their IVD may be further studied for potential use as an efficacious, safe and reversible male contraceptive device [142].

Reversible inhibition of sperm under guidance (RISUG) is another intra-vas technique first tested in rats in 1979 [143]. This technique uses styrene maleic anhydride (SMA) solubilized in dimethylsulfoxide (DMSO) and injected under direct visualization into the vas deferens [62, 144]. Once in the vas deferens, the SMA forms a porous polymer, and Phase II trials in India have shown safety and efficacy through at least 1 year after injection [144]. These initial studies have led to preclinical trials in the United States under the trade name of Vasalgel [62]. Although the possibility for reversal may exist, this technique is likely to be more attractive as a possible alternative to vasectomy than for male contraception in general.

Multipurpose Technologies

The ideal contraceptive would offer the user highly effective birth control with minimal risk. However, additional health benefits would also provide a secondary advantage. Research towards development of multipurpose prevention technologies (MPTs) is new, but may represent the future direction of new contraceptive strategies and investigation. The impetus for MPT development was to protect women against unplanned pregnancy as well as possible infection with HIV or other sexually transmitted pathogens. Currently, condoms and abstinence are the only available methods for STI prevention, and, while these methods are also used for birth control, failure rates with typical use are above 18%. Multiple different strategies are being used to try and provide reliable contraception and STI prevention, particularly HIV prevention. Current research efforts have focused on the concept of a dual protection vaginal ring containing levonorgestrel and an antiretroviral agent; at least three MPT rings are in development [145]. Vaginal gels containing the antiretroviral tenofovir have been shown to decrease HIV transmission, and may be combined with a spermicidal gel for contraception [13, 146]. Similar to the contraceptive ring concept, a vaginal gel with antiretroviral MIV-150 with zinc and levonogestrel in a carrageenan gel was developed by the Population Council [145]. Potential barrier methods include a single-size silicone contraceptive diaphragm (the SILCS diaphragm, recently approved under the name Caya®) which may potentially be combined with active agents, such as antiretroviral gels [145, 147], and the improved Women's Condom; both were developed by PATH and are currently in clinical trials.

Other health benefits associated with specific contraceptive products may be advantageous for users. Mirena® IUS is one of the most effective contraceptive products available to women but it is also used for control of menorrhagia. Development of amenorrhea may be useful in curbing anemia in women who are prone to that condition. Female COCs are often a first-line treatment provided for idiopathic menorrhagia, although this is an "off-label" use. As discussed above, Natazia is a recently approved COC with estradiol valerate and dienogest. The regimen varies the ratio of the hormones to produce contraceptive efficacy with a reduction of heavy menstrual bleeding [20]. A randomized controlled trial of 190 women with prolonged, frequent, or heavy menstrual bleeding showed a mean reduction in menstrual blood loss of -353 ml (-64.2%) compared to placebo -130 ml (-7.8%) ($p<0.001$). The reduction in heavy bleeding may make it an attractive contraceptive choice for women with menorrhagia [21, 148].

Other potential dual benefits that may come from hormonal contraception include previously studied effects, such as improvement in dysmenorrhea, acne and premenstrual dysphoric disorder, as well as newly identified potential benefits [145]. For example, the PRM, CDB-4124, is currently being studied for possible prevention and treatment of breast cancer due to its inhibition of cell proliferation and induction of apoptosis in some mammary tumors [149]. Another promising benefit may be neuroprotection seen in animal studies with the use of some progestins [150, 151].

Despite negative information commonly attributed to pill use, a large study shows that women who use oral contraceptives may live significantly longer than non-users. In a study of 46,112 women observed for up to 39 years in the UK, users of oral contraceptives had significantly lower rates of all deaths from any cause. In particular, they had significantly lower risk of death from all cancers, particularly ovarian, endometrial and colon cancer, as well as from circulatory disease or ischemic heart disease [152]. In this study, the rate of breast cancer was lower in contraceptive users than non-users but the difference was not statistically significant. Other studies confirm the lower rates of ovarian, endometrial and colon cancer in oral contraceptive users [153, 154].

Conclusion

Despite a wide variety of contraceptive products/methods for women, contraceptive needs are not adequately met by currently available methods, as is evidenced by the high rates of unplanned pregnancy in non-users as well as unplanned pregnancy in contraceptive users. Ideally, contraception should be highly effective with minimal side effects, easy to use, fully reversible, and widely available in order to have the greatest impact. Additionally, the burden of pregnancy prevention should not fall solely on the woman's shoulders. Men desire and would benefit from having access to male contraception. Male hormonal contraception has undergone extensive testing, proving efficacy and tolerability. Studies show that medications used currently for treatment of other indications could be combined and used off-label for male contraception. The future of contraception should include male contraceptive options beyond the condom and vasectomy. Another focus of research and advocacy efforts is to expand the availability and use of long-acting reversible contraceptives which have been demonstrated to have extremely low failure rates and have high acceptability/continuation rates [155, 156]. At the time of writing, the American Academy of Pediatrics just published recommendations for expanded use of progestin implants and intrauterine systems for contraception in adolescents, echoing American Congress of Obstetricians and Gynecologists recommendations from 2012 [157, 158]. The coverage of all contraceptive products with no copay in the Affordable Care Act will help to remove the barriers of cost and access for many women. Looking ahead, the research community may also prioritize development of contraception that offers the user dual-benefits. This is particularly important and logical for prevention of STI's, especially HIV globally.

New directions of contraception research could incorporate the concept of 'green contraceptives' [159]. Contraception is already a primary tool for addressing population growth, which consequentially decreases the human burden on the environment [71, 159, 160]. That being said, the entire process of contraceptive design, manufacturing, use of materials, distribution, consumer use and disposal can be approached through an eco-friendly lens [159]. By incorporating more environmentally sustainable practices now while increasing efficacy and availability of family planning globally, the contraceptive community could play a significant role in the preservation of our environment.

With several promising avenues to pursue and the potential to impact STI prevention and environmentally friendly manufacturing practices, novel contraceptive technologies represent a dynamic area of inquiry.

References

[1] Hugon-Rodin, J; Chabbert-Buffet, N; Bouchard, P. The future of women's contraception: stakes and modalities. *Ann N Y Acad Sci*, 2010, 1205, 230-9.

[2] Singh, S; Sedgh, G; Hussain, R. Unintended pregnancy: worldwide levels, trends, and outcomes. *Stud Fam Plann*, 2010, 41(4), 241-50.

[3] Finer, LB; Kost, K. Unintended pregnancy rates at the state level. *Perspect Sex Reprod Health*, 2011, 43(2), 78-87.

[4] Sedgh, G; Singh, S; Hussain, R. Intended and unintended pregnancies worldwide in 2012 and recent trends. *Stud Fam Plann*, 2014, 45(3), 301-14.

[5] Frost, JJ. Darroch, JE. Factors associated with contraceptive choice and inconsistent method use, United States, 2004. *Perspect Sex Reprod Health*, 2008, 40(2), 94-104.

[6] Frost, JJ; Darroch, JE; Remez, L. Improving contraceptive use in the United States. *Issues Brief (Alan Guttmacher Inst)*, 2008(1), 1-8.

[7] Kost, K; et al., Estimates of contraceptive failure from the 2002 National Survey of Family Growth. *Contraception*, 2008, 77(1), 10-21.

[8] Sitruk-Ware, R. Contraception: an international perspective. *Contraception*, 2006, 73(3), p. 215-22.

[9] Nieschlag, E. Clinical trials in male hormonal contraception. *Contraception*, 2010, 82(5), 457-70.

[10] Roth, MY; et al., Acceptability of a transdermal gel-based male hormonal contraceptive in a randomized controlled trial. *Contraception*, 2014, 90(4), 407-12.

[11] Heinemann, K., et al., Attitudes toward male fertility control: results of a multinational survey on four continents. *Hum Reprod*, 2005, 20(2), 549-56.

[12] Goodman, A. The Long Wait for Male Birth Control, in Time. 2008.

[13] Jensen, JT. The future of contraception: innovations in contraceptive agents: tomorrow's hormonal contraceptive agents and their clinical implications. *Am J Obstet Gynecol*, 2011, 205(4 Suppl), S21-5.

[14] Jones, J; Mosher, W; Daniels, K. Current contraceptive use in the United States, 2006-2010, and changes in patterns of use since 1995, 2012, National Health Statistics Reports.

[15] Lievertz, RW. Pharmacology and pharmacokinetics of estrogens. *Am J Obstet Gynecol*, 1987, 156(5), 1289-93.

[16] Helgason, S; et al., Estrogenic potency of oral replacement therapy estimated by the induction of pregnancy zone protein. *Acta Obstet Gynecol Scand*, 1982,61(1), 75-9.

[17] Lidegaard, O; et al., Hormonal contraception and risk of venous thromboembolism: national follow-up study. *BMJ*, 2009, 339, p. b2890.

[18] Dinger, JC; Heinemann, LA; Kuhl-Habich, D. The safety of a drospirenone-containing oral contraceptive: final results from the European Active Surveillance Study on oral contraceptives based on 142,475 women-years of observation. *Contraception*, 2007, 75(5), 344-54.

[19] Lidegaard, O; et al., Venous thrombosis in users of non-oral hormonal contraception: follow-up study, Denmark 2001-10. *BMJ*, 2012, 344, e2990.

[20] Ahrendt, HJ; et al., Bleeding pattern and cycle control with an estradiol-based oral contraceptive: a seven-cycle, randomized comparative trial of estradiol valerate/dienogest and ethinyl estradiol/levonorgestrel. *Contraception*, 2009, 80(5), 436-44.

[21] Jensen, JT; et al., Effective treatment of heavy menstrual bleeding with estradiol valerate and dienogest: a randomized controlled trial. *Obstet Gynecol*, 2011, 117(4), 777-87.

[22] Lello, S. Nomegestrol acetate: pharmacology, safety profile and therapeutic efficacy. *Drugs*, 2010, 70(5), p. 541-59.

[23] Duijkers, IJ; et al., Effects of a monophasic combined oral contraceptive containing nomegestrol acetate and 17 beta-oestradiol on ovarian function in comparison to a monophasic combined oral contraceptive containing drospirenone and ethinylestradiol. *Eur J Contracept Reprod Health Care*, 2010, 15(5), 314-25.

[24] Visser, M; Coelingh Bennink, HJ. Clinical applications for estetrol. *J Steroid Biochem Mol Biol*, 2009, 114(1-2), 85-9.

[25] Chabbert-Buffet, N; et al., Selective progesterone receptor modulators and progesterone antagonists: mechanisms of action and clinical applications. *Hum Reprod Update*, 2005, 11(3), 293-307.

[26] Blithe, DL; et al., Development of the selective progesterone receptor modulator CDB-2914 for clinical indications. *Steroids*, 2003. 68(10-13), 1013-7.

[27] Glasier, AF; et al., Ulipristal acetate versus levonorgestrel for emergency contraception, a randomised non-inferiority trial and meta-analysis. *Lancet*, 2010, 375(9714), 555-62.

[28] Brache, V; et al., Immediate pre-ovulatory administration of 30 mg ulipristal acetate significantly delays follicular rupture. *Hum Reprod*, 2010, 25(9), 2256-63.

[29] Chabbert-Buffet, N; et al., Effects of the progesterone receptor modulator VA2914 in a continuous low dose on the hypothalamic-pituitary-ovarian axis and endometrium in normal women: a prospective, randomized, placebo-controlled trial. *J Clin Endocrinol Metab*, 2007, 92(9), 3582-9.

[30] Brenner, RM. Slayden, OD. Progesterone receptor antagonists and the endometrial antiproliferative effect. *Semin Reprod Med*, 2005, 23(1), 74-81.

[31] Horne, FM; Blithe, DL. Progesterone receptor modulators and the endometrium: changes and consequences. *Hum Reprod Update*, 2007, 13(6), 567-80.

[32] Mutter, GL; et al., The spectrum of endometrial pathology induced by progesterone receptor modulators. *Mod Pathol*, 2008, 21(5), p. 591-8.

[33] Wiegratz, I; et al., Effect of a low-dose contraceptive patch on efficacy, bleeding pattern, and safety: a 1-year, multicenter, open-label, uncontrolled study. *Reprod Sci*, 2014, 21(12), 1518-25.

[34] Sitruk-Ware, RL; et al., Comparison of the impact of vaginal and oral administration of combined hormonal contraceptives on hepatic proteins sensitive to estrogen. *Contraception*, 2007, 75(6), 430-7.

[35] Sitruk-Ware, R. New progestagens for contraceptive use. *Hum Reprod Update*, 2006. 12(2), 169-78.

[36] Sitruk-Ware, R; et al., Nestorone, clinical applications for contraception and HRT. *Steroids*, 2003, 68(10-13), 907-13.

[37] Fraser, IS; et al., An initial pharmacokinetic study with a Metered Dose Transdermal Systemfor delivery of the progestogen Nestorone as a possible future contraceptive. *Contraception*, 2007, 76(6), 432-8.

[38] Brache, V; et al., Effects of a novel estrogen-free, progesterone receptor modulator contraceptive vaginal ring on inhibition of ovulation, bleeding patterns and endometrium in normal women. *Contraception*, 2012, 85(5), 480-8.

[39] Huang, Y; et al., A randomized study on pharmacodynamic effects of vaginal rings delivering the progesterone receptor modulator ulipristal acetate: research for a novel estrogen-free, method of contraception. *Contraception*, 2014,

[40] Massai, MR; et al., Contraceptive efficacy and clinical performance of Nestorone implants in postpartum women. *Contraception*, 2001, 64(6), 369-76.

[41] Sivin, I; et al., Two-year performance of a Nestorone-releasing contraceptive implant: a three-center study of 300 women. *Contraception*, 2004, 69(2), 137-44.

[42] Garza-Flores, J; Hall, PE; Perez-Palacios, G. Long-acting hormonal contraceptives for women. *J Steroid Biochem Mol Biol*, 1991, 40(4-6), 697-704.

[43] Massai, MR; et al., Does meloxicam increase the incidence of anovulation induced by single administration of levonorgestrel in emergency contraception? A pilot study. *Hum Reprod*, 2007, 22(2), 434-9.

[44] Pall, M; Friden, BE; Brannstrom, M. Induction of delayed follicular rupture in the human by the selective COX-2 inhibitor rofecoxib: a randomized double-blind study. *Hum Reprod*, 2001, 16(7), 1323-8.

[45] Jesam, C; et al., Suppression of follicular rupture with meloxicam, a cyclooxygenase-2 inhibitor: potential for emergency contraception. *Hum Reprod*, 2010, 25(2), 368-73.

[46] Han, SJ; et al., Protein kinase B/Akt phosphorylation of PDE3A and its role in mammalian oocyte maturation. *EMBO J*, 2006, 25(24), 5716-25.

[47] Jensen, JT; et al., Evaluation of the phosphodiesterase 3 inhibitor ORG 9935 as a contraceptive in female macaques: initial trials. *Contraception*, 2010, 81(2), 165-71.

[48] Hanna, CB; et al., WEE2 is an oocyte-specific meiosis inhibitor in rhesus macaque monkeys. *Biol Reprod*, 2010, 82(6), 1190-7.

[49] Fan, HY; et al., MAPK3/1 (ERK1/2) in ovarian granulosa cells are essential for female fertility. *Science*, 2009, 324(5929), 938-41.

[50] Bianchi, E; et al., Juno is the egg Izumo receptor and is essential for mammalian fertilization. *Nature*, 2014, 508(7497), 483-7.

[51] Wu, X; et al., Zygote arrest 1 (Zar1) is an evolutionarily conserved gene expressed in vertebrate ovaries. *Biol Reprod*, 2003, 69(3), 861-7.

[52] White, CA; et al., Blocking LIF action in the uterus by using a PEGylated antagonist prevents implantation: a nonhormonal contraceptive strategy. *Proc Natl Acad Sci U S A*, 2007, 104(49), 19357-62.

[53] Sharkey, AM; et al., Novel antiangiogenic agents for use in contraception. *Contraception*, 2005, 71(4), 263-71.

[54] Trussell, J. Contraceptive failure in the United States. *Contraception*, 2011, 83(5), 397-404.
[55] Cleland, K; et al., The efficacy of intrauterine devices for emergency contraception: a systematic review of 35 years of experience. *Hum Reprod*, 2012, 27(7), 1994-2000.
[56] Gemzell-Danielsson, K; Schellschmidt, I; Apter, D. A randomized, phase II study describing the efficacy, bleeding profile, and safety of two low-dose levonorgestrel-releasing intrauterine contraceptive systems and Mirena. *Fertil Steril*, 2012, 97(3), 616-22 e1-3.
[57] An explorative trial to explore the safety, acceptability and vaginal bleeding pattern of three etonogestrel-releasing medicated intrauterine systems. [cited 2014 September 17, 2014]; Available from: http://www.clinicaltrials.gov/ct2/show/results/NCT00967746?term=etonogestrel&rank=13.
[58] Brenner, RM; et al., Intrauterine administration of CDB-2914 (Ulipristal) suppresses the endometrium of rhesus macaques. *Contraception*, 2010, 81(4), p. 336-42.
[59] Brenner, RM; et al., A role for the androgen receptor in the endometrial antiproliferative effects of progesterone antagonists. *Steroids*, 2003, 68(10-13), 1033-9.
[60] Fuhrmann, U., et al., Synthesis and biological activity of a novel, highly potent progesterone receptor antagonist. *J Med Chem*, 2000, 43(26), 5010-6.
[61] Heikinheimo, O; et al., Intrauterine release of progesterone antagonist ZK230211 is feasible and results in novel endometrial effects: a pilot study. *Hum Reprod*, 2007, 22(9), 2515-22.
[62] Kogan, P. Wald, M. Male contraception: history and development. *Urol Clin North Am*, 2014, 41(1), 145-61.
[63] World Health Organization Task Force on Methods for the Regulation of Male, F., Contraceptive efficacy of testosterone-induced azoospermia and oligozoospermia in normal men. *Fertil Steril*, 1996, 65(4), 821-9.
[64] Bebb, RA; et al., Combined administration of levonorgestrel and testosterone induces more rapid and effective suppression of spermatogenesis than testosterone alone: a promising male contraceptive approach. *J Clin Endocrinol Metab*, 1996, 81(2), 757-62.
[65] Lue, Y; et al., Levonorgestrel enhances spermatogenesis suppression by testosterone with greater alteration in testicular gene expression in men. *Biol Reprod*, 2009, 80(3), 484-92.

[66] Bagatell, CJ; et al., Comparison of a gonadotropin releasing-hormone antagonist plus testosterone (T) versus T alone as potential male contraceptive regimens. *J Clin Endocrinol Metab*, 1993, 77(2), 427-32.
[67] Swerdloff, RS; et al., Suppression of spermatogenesis in man induced by Nal-Glu gonadotropin releasing hormone antagonist and testosterone enanthate (TE) is maintained by TE alone. *J Clin Endocrinol Metab*, 1998, 83(10), 3527-33.
[68] Behre, HM; et al., Suppression of spermatogenesis to azoospermia by combined administration of GnRH antagonist and 19-nortestosterone cannot be maintained by this non-aromatizable androgen alone. *Hum Reprod*, 2001, 16(12), 2570-7.
[69] Anderson, RA; Baird, DT. Male contraception. *Endocr Rev*, 2002, 23(6), 735-62.
[70] Wang, C; Swerdloff, RS. Hormonal approaches to male contraception. Curr Opin Urol, 2010, 20(6), 520-4.
[71] Blithe, D. Male contraception: what is on the horizon? *Contraception*, 2008, 78(4 Suppl), S23-7.
[72] Roth, MY; et al., Characteristics associated with suppression of spermatogenesis in a male hormonal contraceptive trial using testosterone and Nestorone((R)) gels. *Andrology*, 2013, 1(6), 899-905.
[73] Ilani, N; et al., Does ethnicity matter in male hormonal contraceptive efficacy? *Asian J Androl*, 2011, 13(4), 579-84.
[74] Kinniburgh, D; et al., Oral desogestrel with testosterone pellets induces consistent suppression of spermatogenesis to azoospermia in both Caucasian and Chinese men. *Hum Reprod*, 2002, 17(6), 1490-501.
[75] Nieschlag, E; et al., Plasma androgen levels in men after oral administration of testosterone or testosterone undecanoate. *Acta Endocrinol (Copenh)*, 1975, 79(2), 366-74.
[76] Westaby, D; et al., Liver damage from long-term methyltestosterone. *Lancet*, 1977, 2(8032), 262-3.
[77] Attardi, BJ., Hild, SA; Reel, JR. Dimethandrolone undecanoate: a new potent orally active androgen with progestational activity. *Endocrinology*, 2006, 147(6), 3016-26.
[78] Surampudi, P; et al., Single, escalating dose pharmacokinetics, safety and food effects of a new oral androgen dimethandrolone undecanoate in man: a prototype oral male hormonal contraceptive. *Andrology*, 2014, 2(4), 579-87.

[79] Kumar, N; et al., The biological activity of 7 alpha-methyl-19-nortestosterone is not amplified in male reproductive tract as is that of testosterone. *Endocrinology*, 1992, 130(6), 3677-83.

[80] Anderson, RA; et al., Evidence for tissue selectivity of the synthetic androgen 7 alpha-methyl-19-nortestosterone in hypogonadal men. *J Clin Endocrinol Metab*, 2003, 88(6), 2784-93.

[81] von Eckardstein, S; et al., A clinical trial of 7 alpha-methyl-19-nortestosterone implants for possible use as a long-acting contraceptive for men. *J Clin Endocrinol Metab*, 2003, 88(11), 5232-9.

[82] Walton, MJ; et al., 7alpha-methyl-19-nortestosterone (MENT) vs testosterone in combination with etonogestrel implants for spermatogenic suppression in healthy men. *J Androl*, 2007, 28(5), 679-88.

[83] Nieschlag, E; Kumar, N; Sitruk-Ware, R. 7alpha-methyl-19-nortestosterone (MENTR): the population council's contribution to research on male contraception and treatment of hypogonadism. *Contraception*, 2013, 87(3), 288-95.

[84] Page, ST; et al., Testosterone gel combined with depomedroxyprogesterone acetate is an effective male hormonal contraceptive regimen and is not enhanced by the addition of a GnRH antagonist. *J Clin Endocrinol Metab*, 2006, 91(11), 4374-80.

[85] Mahabadi, V; et al., Combined transdermal testosterone gel and the progestin nestorone suppresses serum gonadotropins in men. *J Clin Endocrinol Metab*, 2009, 94(7), 2313-20.

[86] Ilani, N; et al., A new combination of testosterone and nestorone transdermal gels for male hormonal contraception. *J Clin Endocrinol Metab*, 2012, 97(10), 3476-86.

[87] Li, JW; Gu, YQ. Predictors for partial suppression of spermatogenesis of hormonal male contraception. *Asian J Androl*, 2008, 10(5), 723-30.

[88] Gu, Y; et al., Multicenter contraceptive efficacy trial of injectable testosterone undecanoate in Chinese men. *J Clin Endocrinol Metab*, 2009, 94(6), 1910-5.

[89] Brady, BM; et al., Depot testosterone with etonogestrel implants result in induction of azoospermia in all men for long-term contraception. *Hum Reprod*, 2004, 19(11), 2658-67.

[90] Mommers, E; et al., Male hormonal contraception: a double-blind, placebo-controlled study. *J Clin Endocrinol Metab*, 2008, 93(7), 2572-80.

[91] Kamischke, A; et al., Intramuscular testosterone undecanoate and norethisterone enanthate in a clinical trial for male contraception. *J Clin Endocrinol Metab*, 2001, 86(1), 303-9.
[92] Nieschlag, E; Zitzmann, M; Kamischke, A. Use of progestins in male contraception. *Steroids*, 2003, 68(10-13), 965-72.
[93] Larkin, A. Male Hormonal Contraceptive Trial Ending Early. 2011 September 3, 2014]; Available from: http://www.conrad.org/news-pressreleases-63.html.
[94] Coutinho, EM; et al., Gossypol blood levels and inhibition of spermatogenesis in men taking gossypol as a contraceptive. A multicenter, international, dose-finding study. *Contraception*, 2000, 61(1), 61-7.
[95] Coutinho, EM. Gossypol: a contraceptive for men. *Contraception*, 2002, 65(4), 259-63.
[96] Cheng, CY; et al., Two new male contraceptives exert their effects by depleting germ cells prematurely from the testis. *Biol Reprod*, 2001, 65(2), 449-61.
[97] Vickery, BH. Non-steroidal interference with male fertility. *Adv Contracept*, 1986, 2(1), 1-30.
[98] Hild, SA; et al., Development of l-CDB-4022 as a nonsteroidal male oral contraceptive: induction and recovery from severe oligospermia in the adult male cynomolgus monkey (Macaca fascicularis). *Endocrinology*, 2007, 148(4), 1784-96.
[99] Mruk, DD; et al., A male contraceptive targeting germ cell adhesion. *Nat Med*, 2006, 12(11), 1323-8.
[100] Mok, KW; et al., Adjudin, a potential male contraceptive, exerts its effects locally in the seminiferous epithelium of mammalian testes. *Reproduction*, 2011, 141(5), 571-80.
[101] Cheng, CY; et al., Adjudin disrupts spermatogenesis via the action of some unlikely partners: Eps8, Arp2/3 complex, drebrin E, PAR6 and 14-3-3. *Spermatogenesis*, 2011, 1(4), 291-297.
[102] Tash, JS; et al., A novel potent indazole carboxylic acid derivative blocks spermatogenesis and is contraceptive in rats after a single oral dose. *Biol Reprod*, 2008, 78(6), 1127-38.
[103] Wolgemuth, DJ; Chung, SS. Retinoid signaling during spermatogenesis as revealed by genetic and metabolic manipulations of retinoic acid receptor alpha. *Soc Reprod Fertil Suppl*, 2007, 63, 11-23.

[104] Anderson, EL; et al., Stra8 and its inducer, retinoic acid, regulate meiotic initiation in both spermatogenesis and oogenesis in mice. *Proc Natl Acad Sci U S A*, 2008, 105(39), 14976-80.

[105] Coulston, F; Beyler, AL; Drobeck, HP. The biologic actions of a new series of bis(dichloroacetyl) diamines. *Toxicol Appl Pharmacol*, 1960, 2, 715-31.

[106] Heller, CG; Moore, DJ; Paulsen, CA. Suppression of spermatogenesis and chronic toxicity in men by a new series of bis(dichloroacetyl) diamines. *Toxicol Appl Pharmacol*, 1961, 3, 1-11.

[107] Amory, JK; et al., Suppression of spermatogenesis by bisdichloroacetyldiamines is mediated by inhibition of testicular retinoic acid biosynthesis. *J Androl*, 2011, 32(1), 111-9.

[108] Hogarth, CA; et al., Suppression of Stra8 expression in the mouse gonad by WIN 18,446. *Biol Reprod*, 2011, 84(5), 957-65.

[109] Hogarth, CA; et al., Turning a spermatogenic wave into a tsunami: synchronizing murine spermatogenesis using WIN 18,446. *Biol Reprod*, 2013, 88(2), 40.

[110] Chung, SS; et al., Oral administration of a retinoic Acid receptor antagonist reversibly inhibits spermatogenesis in mice. *Endocrinology*, 2011, 152(6), 2492-502.

[111] Schulze, GE; et al., BMS-189453, a novel retinoid receptor antagonist, is a potent testicular toxin. *Toxicol Sci*, 2001, 59(2), 297-308.

[112] Chung, SS; Wang, X; Wolgemuth, DJ. Expression of retinoic acid receptor alpha in the germline is essential for proper cellular association and spermiogenesis during spermatogenesis. *Development*, 2009, 136(12), 2091-100.

[113] Shang, E; et al., The first bromodomain of Brdt, a testis-specific member of the BET sub-family of double-bromodomain-containing proteins, is essential for male germ cell differentiation. *Development*, 2007, 134(19), 3507-15.

[114] Gaucher, J; et al., Bromodomain-dependent stage-specific male genome programming by Brdt. *EMBO J*, 2012, 31(19), 3809-20.

[115] Aston, KI; et al., Evaluation of 172 candidate polymorphisms for association with oligozoospermia or azoospermia in a large cohort of men of European descent. *Hum Reprod*, 2010, 25(6), 1383-97.

[116] Matzuk, MM; et al., Small-molecule inhibition of BRDT for male contraception. *Cell*, 2012, 150(4), 673-84.

[117] Lishko, PV; et al., The control of male fertility by spermatozoan ion channels. *Annu Rev Physiol*, 2012, 74, 453-75.

[118] Navarro, B; Kirichok, Y; Clapham, DE. KSper, a pH-sensitive K+ current that controls sperm membrane potential. *Proc Natl Acad Sci U S A*, 2007, 104(18), 7688-92.
[119] Qi, H; et al., All four CatSper ion channel proteins are required for male fertility and sperm cell hyperactivated motility. *Proc Natl Acad Sci U S A*, 2007, 104(4), 1219-23.
[120] Li, H; et al., Immunization of male mice with B-cell epitopes in transmembrane domains of CatSper1 inhibits fertility. *Fertil Steril*, 2012, 97(2), 445-52.
[121] Carlson, AE; et al., Pharmacological targeting of native CatSper channels reveals a required role in maintenance of sperm hyperactivation. *PLoS One*, 2009, 4(8), e6844.
[122] Hunter, RH. Sperm release from oviduct epithelial binding is controlled hormonally by peri-ovulatory graafian follicles. *Mol Reprod Dev*, 2008, 75(1), 167-74.
[123] Wang, D; et al., A new sperm-specific Na+/H+ exchanger required for sperm motility and fertility. *Nat Cell Biol*, 2003, 5(12), 1117-22.
[124] Wang, D; et al., A sperm-specific Na+/H+ exchanger (sNHE) is critical for expression and in vivo bicarbonate regulation of the soluble adenylyl cyclase (sAC). *Proc Natl Acad Sci U S A*, 2007, 104(22), 9325-30.
[125] Sanchez, G; et al., The Na,K-ATPase alpha4 isoform from humans has distinct enzymatic properties and is important for sperm motility. *Mol Hum Reprod*, 2006, 12(9), 565-76.
[126] Woo, AL; James, PF; Lingrel, JB. Sperm motility is dependent on a unique isoform of the Na,K-ATPase. *J Biol Chem*, 2000, 275(27), 20693-9.
[127] Woo, AL; James, PF; Lingrel, JB. Roles of the Na,K-ATPase alpha4 isoform and the Na+/H+ exchanger in sperm motility. *Mol Reprod Dev*, 2002, 62(3), 348-56.
[128] Jimenez, T; et al., Na,K-ATPase alpha4 isoform is essential for sperm fertility. *Proc Natl Acad Sci U S A*, 2011, 108(2), 644-9.
[129] Thundathil, JC; Anzar, M; Buhr, MM. Na+/K+ATPase as a signaling molecule during bovine sperm capacitation. *Biol Reprod*, 2006, 75(3), 308-17.
[130] Newton, LD; et al., Na+/K+ATPase regulates sperm capacitation through a mechanism involving kinases and redistribution of its testis-specific isoform. *Mol Reprod Dev*, 2010, 77(2), 136-48.
[131] Woo, AL; James, PF; Lingrel, JB. Characterization of the fourth alpha isoform of the Na,K-ATPase. *J Membr Biol*, 1999, 169(1), 39-44.

[132] Konrad, L; et al., Cardiotonic *steroids* trigger non-classical testosterone signaling in Sertoli cells via the alpha4 isoform of the sodium pump. *Biochim Biophys Acta*, 2011, 1813(12), 2118-24.

[133] Clausen, MJ; Nissen, P; Poulsen, H. The pumps that fuel a sperm's journey. *Biochem Soc Trans*, 2011, 39(3), 741-5.

[134] Nomura, M; Vacquier, VD. Proteins associated with soluble adenylyl cyclase in sea urchin sperm flagella. *Cell Motil Cytoskeleton*, 2006, 63(9), 582-90.

[135] Ickowicz, D; Finkelstein, M; Breitbart, H. Mechanism of sperm capacitation and the acrosome reaction: role of protein kinases. *Asian J Androl*, 2012, 14(6), 816-21.

[136] Battistone, MA; et al., Functional human sperm capacitation requires both bicarbonate-dependent PKA activation and down-regulation of Ser/Thr phosphatases by Src family kinases. *Mol Hum Reprod*, 2013, 19(9), 570-80.

[137] Kwon, WS; et al., Vasopressin effectively suppresses male fertility. PLoS One, 2013,8(1), p. e54192.

[138] de Lamirande, E; O'Flaherty, C. Sperm activation: role of reactive oxygen species and kinases. *Biochim Biophys Acta*, 2008, 1784(1), 106-15.

[139] Lee, HY. Experimental studies on reversible vas occlusion by intravasal thread. *Fertil Steril*, 1969. 20(5), 735-44.

[140] Song, L; et al., A phase II randomized controlled trial of a novel male contraception, an intra-vas device. *Int J Androl*, 2006, 29(4), 489-95.

[141] Huang, XB; et al., Initial studies on a novel filtering-type intra-vas device in male dogs. *Contraception*, 2010, 81(4), 350-4.

[142] Chen, ZL; et al., The contraceptive effect of a novel filtering-type nano-copper complex/polymer composites intra-vas device on male animals. *Int J Androl*, 2010, 33(6), 810-7.

[143] Misro, M; et al., Injectable non-occlusive chemical contraception in the male-I. *Contraception*, 1979, 20(5), 467-73.

[144] Guha, SK; et al., Phase II clinical trial of a vas deferens injectable contraceptive for the male. *Contraception*, 1997, 56(4), 245-50.

[145] Sitruk-Ware, R; Nath, A; Mishell, DR. Jr. Contraception technology: past, present and future. *Contraception*, 2013, 87(3), 319-30.

[146] Abdool Karim, Q; et al., Effectiveness and safety of tenofovir gel, an antiretroviral microbicide, for the prevention of HIV infection in women. *Science*, 2010, 329(5996), 1168-74.

[147] Schwartz, JL; et al., SILCS diaphragm: postcoital testing of a new single-size contraceptive device. *Contraception*, 2008, 78(3), 237-44.
[148] Nappi, RE; Serrani, M; Jensen, JT. Noncontraceptive benefits of the estradiol valerate/dienogest combined oral contraceptive: a review of the literature. *Int J Womens Health*, 2014, 6, 711-8.
[149] Wiehle, R; et al., CDB-4124, a progesterone receptor modulator, inhibits mammary carcinogenesis by suppressing cell proliferation and inducing apoptosis. *Cancer Prev Res (Phila)*, 2011, 4(3), 414-24.
[150] Liu, L; et al., Clinically relevant progestins regulate neurogenic and neuroprotective responses in vitro and in vivo. *Endocrinology*, 2010, 151(12), 5782-94.
[151] Hussain, R; et al., Progesterone and Nestorone facilitate axon remyelination: a role for progesterone receptors. *Endocrinology*, 2011, 152(10), 3820-31.
[152] Hannaford, PC; et al., Mortality among contraceptive pill users: cohort evidence from Royal College of General Practitioners' Oral Contraception Study. *BMJ*, 2010, 340, p. c927.
[153] Bosetti, C; et al., Oral contraceptives and colorectal cancer risk: a systematic review and meta-analysis. *Hum Reprod Update*, 2009, 15(5), 489-98.
[154] National Cancer Institute. Oral Contraceptives and Cancer Risk. November 28, 2014]; Available from: http://www.cancer.gov/cancertopics/factsheet/risk/oral-contraceptives.
[155] Peipert, JF; et al., Continuation and satisfaction of reversible contraception. *Obstet Gynecol*, 2011, 117(5), 1105-13.
[156] McNicholas, C; et al., The Contraceptive CHOICE Project Round Up: What We Did and What We Learned. Clin *Obstet Gynecol*, 2014, 57(4), 635-43.
[157] Ott, MA; Sucato, GS; Committee On, A. Contraception for Adolescents. *Pediatrics*, 2014,
[158] Committee on Adolescent Health Care Long-Acting Reversible Contraception Working Group, T.A.C.o.O. and Gynecologists, Committee opinion no. 539: adolescents and long-acting reversible contraception: implants and intrauterine devices. *Obstet Gynecol*, 2012, 120(4), 983-8.
[159] Moore, K; et al., A greenprint for sustainable contraceptive research and development. *Contraception*, 2013, 87(3), 347-51.

[160] Page, ST; Amory, JK; Bremner, WJ. Advances in male contraception. *Endocr Rev*, 2008, 29(4), 465-93.

[161] Ko, JK[1]; Huang, VW; Li, RH; Yeung, WS; Ho, PC; Chiu, PC. An in vitro study of the effect of mifepristone and ulipristal acetate on human sperm functions. *Andrology*, 2014, 2, 868-74.

Index

A

acid, 101, 114, 115
acne, 53, 72, 75, 76, 105
acrosome, 103, 117
adenomyosis, 50
adhesion, 66, 114
adolescent female, 18
adolescents, vii, 12, 17, 18, 19, 20, 21, 27, 34, 48, 55, 76, 78, 81, 106, 118
adverse effects, 3
adverse event, 11, 26
advocacy, 106
AFM, 35
Africa, 3
African American women, 21
age, 6, 10, 17, 18, 23, 33, 76, 82, 86, 89, 92
agonist, 94
AIDS, 60
allergy, 49
amenorrhea, 46, 72, 75, 92, 97, 105
ampulla, 102
anatomy, 74
anchoring, 101
androgen(s), 53, 65, 98, 111, 112, 113
anemia, 73, 105
antiphospholipid syndrome, 11
anxiety, 76
apoptosis, 105, 118
artery, 9
assessment, 82
atherosclerotic plaque, 51
atrophy, 72, 97
attitudes, 93
awareness, 25, 28, 44, 46, 49, 58

B

back pain, 45, 75
bacterial infection, 41
barriers, 3, 6, 15, 18, 27, 28, 30, 106
behaviors, 71
benefits, viii, 3, 46, 47, 51, 53, 55, 74, 91, 92, 104, 105, 106, 118
benign, 76
bicarbonate, 116, 117
binding globulin, 52, 53, 65, 66
bioavailability, 12, 98, 99
biological activity, 111, 113
biosynthesis, 101, 115
birth control, 2, 7, 8, 10, 11, 19, 20, 22, 23, 42, 43, 93, 95, 104
birth rate, 17, 19, 27
births, vii, 17, 39
black women, 21, 22
bleeding, 42, 43, 50, 53, 54, 61, 62, 65, 72, 73, 74, 75, 76, 77, 78, 80, 85, 87, 92, 93, 94, 95, 105, 108, 109, 111
blood, 8, 25, 52, 65, 83, 105, 114
blood clot, 8

blood pressure, 52, 65
blood vessels, 83
BMI, 9
body fluid, 25
bone(s), 40, 75
breast cancer, 76, 78, 105
breast feeding, 52
breast milk, 25
breastfeeding, 3, 48, 59, 76, 95

C

calcium, 102
canals, 41
cancer, 85, 89, 105, 118
candidates, 7, 55, 69, 74, 76, 82, 84, 85, 100
carbohydrate(s), 51, 52, 65
carbohydrate metabolism, 51, 65
carboxylic acid, 100, 114
carcinogenesis, 118
carcinoma, 84, 85
cardiovascular disease(s), 9, 51, 63
Catholic Church, 22
Catholics, 22
Caucasians, 98
CDC, 10, 55, 69, 73
cell culture, 67
cell differentiation, 115
cervicitis, 72
cervix, 40, 41, 48
cesarean section, 73
chemical, 47, 87, 117
Chicago, 29
childcare, 2
children, 2, 19, 23, 40
China, 103
Chinese women, 40
chlamydia, 47, 48
cholesterol, 52, 66
Christians, 23
circulation, 32
clinical application, 108, 109
clinical trials, 53, 69, 80, 85, 95, 97, 99, 100, 104
colon cancer, 105
colorectal cancer, 118
communication, 8, 19, 21, 27, 31, 102
community(s), 23, 41, 93, 106
compliance, viii, 6, 18, 55, 70, 74, 82, 88, 91, 95
complications, 6, 7, 10, 68, 72, 76, 83, 84, 87, 93, 103
compounds, 42, 100
conception, 22, 58, 61
congestive heart failure, 102
Congress, 15, 21, 27, 28, 36, 106
consent, 20
consumption, 46
contaminant, 42
contraceptives, 4, 5, 10, 11, 12, 23, 25, 49, 51, 52, 55, 56, 59, 60, 61, 62, 63, 64, 65, 66, 67, 68, 70, 82, 105, 106, 108, 109, 110, 114, 118
controlled trials, 66
controversial, 9, 23
conversations, 19
copolymer, 75
copper, 13, 71, 72, 74, 79, 103, 117
cortisol, 52
cost, 4, 5, 6, 13, 14, 15, 18, 27, 44, 47, 51, 68, 106
counsel, 55, 85
counseling, 4, 12, 21, 24, 26, 74, 86, 87
country of origin, 23
cox-2 inhibitor, 96
culture, 6, 23
cycles, 46, 53, 61, 95, 96
cyclooxygenase, 96, 110
cytomegalovirus, 48

D

deaths, 24, 31, 105
deficiency, 32
Denmark, 108
Department of Health and Human Services, 4, 21, 31
derivatives, 100, 102
developed countries, 2
developing countries, 2

developing nations, 2
DHS, 29
diabetes, 6, 52, 75, 76
diamines, 115
diaphragm, 41, 47, 59, 104, 118
dimethylsulfoxide, 104
discomfort, 26, 47, 54, 71
diseases, 36
disorder, 10, 74, 105
distribution, 9, 106
District of Columbia, 20
diversity, 100
dizziness, 75
DNA, 58
dogs, 103, 117
dosage, 26
dosing, 53, 55, 60, 62
down-regulation, 117
drug safety, 8, 31
drugs, 12, 32, 101, 102, 103
dyslipidemia, 76
dysmenorrhea, 72, 73, 75, 76, 105
epidemiologic, 65
epididymis, 103
epididymitis, 68, 87
epilepsy, 6, 11
epithelium, 100, 114
epitopes, 116
ester, 99
estriol, 93
estrogen, 6, 7, 8, 9, 11, 26, 43, 45, 50, 51, 52, 53, 54, 61, 93, 94, 109
ethics, 35
ethnic groups, 33
ethnicity, 14, 17, 98, 112
ethylene, 75
Europe, vii, 41, 94
evidence, 12, 23, 25, 32, 44, 52, 54, 67, 73, 88, 96, 103, 118
excision, 83, 84, 86
exercise, 28
exposure, 25, 95
expulsion, 72, 73, 84
extracts, 42

E

echoing, 106
ectopic pregnancy, 74, 79
education, 4, 6, 11, 13, 18, 21, 23, 26, 27, 28, 70
egg, 110
Egypt, 59
ejaculation, 44
electrocautery, 87
eligibility criteria, 74
emergency, 23, 28, 54, 67, 74, 94, 97, 102, 108, 110, 111
employers, 28
empowerment, 24
endocrinology, 31
endometrial hyperplasia, 73, 78
endometriosis, 50, 73, 79
endometritis, 73
energy, 84
environment, 72, 106
enzymes, 92

F

fallopian tubes, 84
families, 13, 87
family history, 52
family planning, 3, 13, 16, 18, 20, 24, 29, 30, 33, 34, 36, 57, 58, 59, 67, 81, 87, 93, 106
fat, 98
fear, 3, 26, 76
federal funds, 16
federal law, 20
feedback inhibition, 98
Female Devices, 97
female partner, 67
femininity, 23
fertility, 23, 33, 40, 44, 46, 49, 50, 51, 58, 68, 69, 70, 72, 81, 86, 87, 93, 101, 102, 103, 107, 110, 114, 115, 116, 117
fertilization, viii, 42, 54, 68, 72, 91, 96, 102, 110
fetus, 25

fever, 25
fibrinogen, 9
fibrosis, 76
films, 48
financial, 2, 4, 6, 13, 15, 18, 27
financial resources, 4
flora, 72
fluid, 44, 58, 103
foams, 48
follicle(s), 50, 96
Food and Drug Administration (FDA), 8, 31, 42, 43, 71, 94, 99, 100
formation, 87
funding, 16, 27, 28

G

gastroenteritis, 51
gel, 48, 59, 60, 93, 95, 99, 104, 107, 113, 117
gene expression, 111
general anesthesia, 68, 83
genes, 92, 96
genome, 101, 115
germ cells, 114
gestational age, 24
gestational diabetes, 52, 65
gland, 57
glucose tolerance, 52
God, 23
gonorrhea, 47, 48, 59
governments, 3
graafian follicle, 116
grants, 42, 93
granulomas, 68
growth, 54, 69, 74, 84, 96
growth factor, 96
guidelines, 70, 73, 89
gynecologist, 41

H

haemostasis, 31
headache, 32, 72, 75
health, vii, viii, 2, 3, 15, 16, 18, 19, 20, 22, 26, 30, 31, 32, 33, 34, 35, 36, 40, 51, 69, 70, 76, 82, 91, 92, 93, 104, 105
Health and Human Services, 39
health care, 3, 15, 18, 32, 34, 36, 76
health care system, 3, 34
health insurance, 82
health risks, 26
heart attack, 64
heart disease, 6, 105
hematoma(s), 68, 87
hemorrhage, 25
hemorrhagic stroke, 52
hepatotoxicity, 98
heterogeneity, 46
high density lipoprotein, 66
high school, 18
higher education, 82
hirsutism, 65
Hispanics, 21
histone, 101
history, 11, 40, 42, 55, 56, 74, 82, 111
HIV, vii, 12, 44, 48, 58, 59, 60, 86, 92, 104, 106, 117
horizontal transmission, 25
hormone(s), 6, 8, 11, 12, 50, 51, 56, 58, 61, 62, 65, 66, 75, 80, 98, 99, 105, 112
hospitalization, 24, 82
HPV, 48
human immunodeficiency virus (HIV/ HIV-1),vii, 12, 44, 48, 58, 59, 60, 86, 92, 104, 106, 117
Hunter, 116
husband, 3
hypertension, 7, 31, 52, 55, 75, 76
hypogonadism, 113
hypothalamus, 46, 49, 98
hysterectomy, 86

I

iconography, 55
idiopathic, 105
implant placement, 84

implants, 18, 76, 95, 97, 98, 99, 106, 110, 113, 118
impotence, 87
improvements, viii, 28, 91, 92
in vitro, 42, 67, 102, 118, 119
in vivo, 116, 118
incidence, 47, 72, 110
income, 4, 6, 13, 14, 15, 16, 18, 26, 27
increased access, 2, 16
India, 104
individuals, 15, 44, 92, 98
inducer, 115
induction, 105, 108, 113, 114
industry, 100
infants, 24
infarction, 51, 64
infection, 25, 41, 47, 59, 60, 68, 72, 73, 86, 87, 104, 117
inferiority, 67, 108
infertility, 44, 100, 101, 102
influenza virus, 24
infrastructure, 3
inhibition, 62, 65, 94, 95, 96, 101, 104, 105, 109, 114, 115
inhibitor, 96, 101, 110
initiation, 74, 101, 115
injections, 95, 99
insertion, 4, 26, 41, 71, 72, 73, 75, 76, 78, 79, 84
insulin, 52
integrity, 60
intercourse, 3, 13, 17, 43, 44, 45, 47, 48, 49, 54, 74, 97
interference, 94, 114
intrauterine contraceptive device, 60, 79
investment, 3, 5, 93
involution, 73, 82
ion channels, 102, 115
Islam, 35
Israel, 35, 41

J

Japan, 41, 56

K

K^+, 102, 116

L

labeling, 77
lactation, 76
laparoscopic surgery, 83
laparoscopy, 82, 83, 84
laparotomy, 82, 83, 84
laws, 83
LDL, 52
lead, 40, 46, 50, 54, 75, 101
Lebanon, 23
legislation, 28
leiomyoma, 78
lesions, 94
ligand, 101
lipids, 52
liver, 76, 93
liver disease, 76
local anesthesia, 84
Long acting reversible contraception, 70
longitudinal study, 58, 60
low risk, 11, 49
lupus, 6, 11

M

male animals, 101, 117
male contraception, 67
male hormonal contraception, 106, 113
malignancy, 94
management, 4, 33, 36, 71
manufacturing, 106
marital status, 46
marriage, 21, 22, 23, 35
married couples, 5, 86
married women, 2, 3
Mars, 32
Maryland, 29
mass, 40, 42
materials, 40, 106

matrix, 53
Mauritania, 23
measurement, 46
median, 69
Medicaid, 5, 16, 18, 20, 33, 34, 57
medical, vii, 1, 6, 7, 15, 26, 27, 33, 35, 41, 48, 55, 82, 85, 86, 98
medical care, 15
medical history, 82
medication, 11, 12, 42, 46, 51, 55, 96, 101
medicine, 30, 31, 32, 35
meiosis, 96, 101, 110
mellitus, 65
menorrhagia, 71, 72, 73, 78, 94, 105
menstrual cycles, 50
mercury, 40
meta-analysis, 64, 67, 79, 108, 118
metabolism, 31
metabolized, 93
metals, 41
Mexico, 29
mice, 96, 102, 103, 115, 116
micrograms, 43, 75
migraine headache, 11
migraines, 11, 75
migration, 76
minority groups, 4, 6
minors, 20
miscarriage(s), vii, 40, 73
misconceptions, 6, 23, 77
Missouri, 6
models, 42, 97, 100, 101, 102
molecules, viii, 91, 96
mood swings, 75
morbidity, 24, 25, 84, 85
mortality, 24, 25, 29, 34, 85
motivation, 46, 58
mucosa, 47, 48
mucous membrane(s), 25
mucus, 45, 50, 52, 61, 94
Muslims, 23
mutagenesis, 101
mutations, 6, 85, 89, 101, 102
myeloproliferative disorders, 11
myocardial infarction, 9, 51, 63, 64

N

Na^+, 102, 116
National Institutes of Health, 1, 31, 39, 91
National Survey, 5, 30, 34, 44, 70, 92, 107
nausea, 54
neonates, 24
neuroprotection, 105
New England, 30, 31, 32, 36, 58-61, 63, 65
New Zealand, 63, 78
nickel, 41, 84
nonsmokers, 51
North America, 24, 87
NSAIDs, 72

O

obesity, 7, 31, 75
occlusion, 5, 83, 84, 85, 86, 89, 117
oligomenorrhea, 72, 75
oligospermia, 69, 98, 114
oligozoospermia, 98, 101, 111, 115
oocyte, 58, 96, 102, 110
oogenesis, 101, 115
opt out, 16
orchitis, 68
organs, 51, 83
outpatient, 83, 84, 86, 89
ovarian cancer, 85, 89
ovarian cysts, 65, 72
ovaries, 42, 110
overweight, 9, 31
oviduct, 102, 116
ovulation, viii, 9, 42, 44-46, 49, 52, 53, 54, 57, 58, 65, 67, 75, 76, 91, 93-96, 109
ovum, 23, 44, 72

P

pain, 26, 45, 72, 73, 75, 79, 85, 87, 94
palpation, 76
parental consent, 20
parental involvement, 20
parents, 19, 20, 27

participants, 12, 26, 66, 76, 95, 99
pathogens, 104
pathology, 84, 94, 109
pathways, 102
peer influence, 23
pelvic inflammatory disease, 47, 59, 72, 78, 86
pelvis, 83
penis, 40
perforation, 72, 73, 84
peritoneal cavity, 86
permeability, 60
permission, 20
permit, 23, 94
personal communication, 101
personal views, 24
pH, 116
pharmacokinetics, 66, 98, 107, 112
pharmacology, 33, 108
Philadelphia, 56
phosphorylation, 103, 110
physicians, 50, 54, 55
physiology, 42
pigs, 42
pilot study, 67, 110, 111
placebo, 11, 48, 94, 96, 99, 105, 109, 113
plants, 40, 100
policy, 20, 23, 33, 39
politics, 33
polydimethylsiloxane, 71
polymer composite material, 103
polymer composites, 117
polymorphisms, 101, 115
polyps, 73
polyurethane, 48
polyvinyl alcohol, 103
POPs, 52
population, 6, 9, 10, 11, 12, 20, 24, 29, 35, 46, 70, 86, 88, 92, 99, 106, 113
population growth, 92, 106
potential benefits, 100, 105
poverty, 13
poverty line, 13
preservation, 106
prevention, viii, 21, 49, 59, 60, 68, 70, 71, 73, 77, 85, 86, 89, 91, 99, 104-106, 117
progesterone, 8, 11, 27, 42, 45, 49, 50, 51, 54, 57, 94, 97, 102, 108, 109, 111, 118
progestins, 8, 94, 99, 105, 114, 118
programming, 115
project, 6, 18, 33, 34, 76
prolactin, 46
proliferation, 105, 118
protease inhibitors, 12
protection, 44, 51, 55, 73, 86, 92, 104
protein kinases, 102, 117
proteins, 92, 96, 103, 109, 115, 116
Protestants, 22
prototype, 112
public health, 9, 11, 30, 33, 36, 37
pumps, 102, 117

R

race, 14, 17
reactions, 53
reactive oxygen, 117
receptacle, 40
receptors, 101, 118
recognition, 101
recommendations, 27, 55, 106
recovery, 25, 68, 84, 86, 101, 114
redistribution, 116
reform, 15, 16, 33
regression, 78
regulations, 20
religion, 22, 23, 24, 28, 34, 35
remyelination, 118
reproduction, 33, 35, 36, 37, 92
reproductive age, 2, 3, 10, 11, 12, 13, 24, 25, 28, 70, 78, 81, 95
reproductive organs, 23
requirements, 71, 83
researchers, 26
resistance, 24, 98
resources, 34, 87
response, 40, 61, 72, 84, 99
restoration, 72
RH, 116, 119

rhythm, 22, 23
rights, 35
rings, 56, 67, 95, 97, 104, 109
risk(s), viii, 2, 7-11, 24, 25, 31, 41, 43, 47, 48, 51, 52, 53, 55, 57, 60, 63, 64, 65, 66, 68, 72-74, 76, 82, 83, 85, 86, 87, 88, 89, 91, 93, 94, 98, 100, 104, 105, 108, 118
risk factors, 11, 52, 60, 64
root, 42
rubber, 40, 83
rules, 45, 46

S

safety, 6, 12, 43, 60, 61, 62, 65, 68, 93, 98, 104, 108, 109, 111, 112, 117
salts, 72
scope, 24
second generation, 9
secretion, 49, 57, 98
seizure, 12, 75
selectivity, 113
semen, 25, 68, 87, 103
sensation, 54
sensitivity, 20, 99
sepsis, 73
Sertoli cells, 100, 117
serum, 66, 96, 99, 113
services, 13, 15, 18, 20, 24, 34, 73, 77, 83, 87
sex, 17, 19, 20, 21, 42, 51, 52, 53, 58, 59, 65, 66
sex hormones, 42
sex steroid, 42, 51
sexism, 24
sexual activity, 13, 17, 20, 21, 49
sexual behavior, 21
sexual behaviour, 58
sexual contact, 25
sexual intercourse, 22, 58
sexually transmitted diseases, 59
sexually transmitted infections, 6, 44, 73, 92
showing, 97, 98, 102
sickle cell, 6, 11, 75
side effects, vii, viii, 23, 26, 40, 46, 47, 50, 51, 54, 68, 72, 74, 75, 77, 79, 81, 92, 94, 95, 96, 98, 100, 106
signs, 44
silicon, 103
silkworm, 41
silver, 41
Sinai, 58
skin, 25, 53, 75
smoking, 7, 52, 55
sodium, 102, 117
solution, 18
Somalia, 23
South Asia, 3
species, 100, 117
speculation, 93
spending, 33
sperm, viii, 27, 40, 44, 45, 47, 48, 49, 57, 68, 72, 91, 94, 98, 99, 100, 101, 102, 103, 104, 116, 117, 119
sperm function, 94, 119
spermatogenesis, 98, 99, 101, 111, 112, 113, 114, 115
spermicide, 23, 47
spontaneous abortion, 25, 83
Spring, 8, 16, 31
state(s), 15, 16, 17, 18, 20, 27, 33, 44, 49, 56, 83, 107
statistics, 17, 22, 30
steel, 84
sterile, 42, 72, 101
Sterilization, 81, 82, 83, 86, 87, 88, 89, 90
steroids, 61, 117
stroke, 6, 9, 11, 51, 52, 63, 64
styrene, 104
success rate, 103
Sudan, 23
Sun, 67, 89
suppository, 40
suppression, 52, 53, 95, 98, 99, 111-113
Supreme Court, 16, 20
surgical intervention, 25
symptoms, 44, 45, 72, 75
synthesis, 33, 96

T

tamoxifen, 78
target, 26, 96, 101, 102
Task Force, 67, 79, 111
techniques, 4, 23, 45, 46, 83, 84, 86, 88, 89
technology(s), vii, 26, 28, 84, 86, 104, 106, 117
teens, 17, 19, 20, 28, 34
temperature, 45, 46, 58
testing, 99, 106, 118
testis, 101, 114, 115, 116
testosterone, 27, 98, 99, 111-114, 117
therapeutic use, 101
therapy, 12, 108
thrombosis, 8, 9, 10, 11, 51, 94, 108
thyroid, 65
tissue, 84, 94, 113
titanium, 83, 84
toxicity, 100, 101, 115
toxin, 115
training, 46, 49, 76
transcripts, 97
transmission, 12, 25, 40, 47-49, 58-60, 104
transportation, 28
treatment, 42, 50, 54, 73, 78, 94, 95, 99, 105, 106, 108, 113
trial, 12, 54, 59, 62, 66, 67, 74, 76, 79, 93, 94, 97, 98, 99, 103, 105, 107, 108, 109, 111, 112, 113, 114, 117
trichomonas, 47, 48
triglycerides, 52
tubal ligation, 5, 84, 86, 87
tumors, 105
Turkey, 23
type 2 diabetes, 65
tyrosine, 103

U

UK, vii, 105
ultrasound, 72
uninsured, 15, 16, 26
United Nations, 2, 29, 69
United States (USA), vii, viii, 1, 2, 3, 4, 5, 11, 14, 17, 21, 22, 23, 25, 28, 29, 30, 36, 43, 49, 56, 57, 65, 68, 69, 71, 76, 77, 79, 82, 84, 87, 89, 92, 93, 94, 104, 107, 111
Unmet Contraceptive Needs, 24
unplanned pregnancies, 2
urethane, 103
urinary tract infection, 48, 59, 60
urine, 42
uterine fibroids, 73, 94
uterus, 41, 73, 110

V

vaccinations, 24, 25
vagina, 48
vaginitis, 54, 75
variables, 63
vas deferens, 68, 86, 103, 104, 117
vasectomy, viii, 5, 13, 68, 69, 70, 82, 86, 87, 89, 90, 91, 93, 97, 103, 104, 106
vasopressin, 103
vasovagal syncope, 85
viruses, 24, 25

W

Washington, 33, 34, 39, 69
weight gain, 75
West Africa, 24, 36
World Health Organization (WHO), 25, 29, 36, 68, 69, 74, 79, 95, 111

Y

young adults, 11, 12
young women, 4, 18, 20, 27, 60, 64

Z

zinc, 104